Contact Lenses
for Pre- and
Post-Surgery

Contact Lenses for Pre- and Post-Surgery

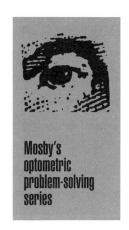

Mosby's optometric problem-solving series

Edited by

Michael G. Harris
OD, JD, MS

Associate Dean
Clinical Professor
Chief, Contact Lens Clinic
School of Optometry
University of California, Berkeley
Berkeley, California

Series Editor
Richard London
MA, OD, FAAO

Diplomate in Binocular Vision and Perception
Pediatric and Rehabilitative Optometry
Oakland, California

*with 88 illustrations
and 32 color plates*

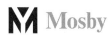 Mosby

St. Louis Baltimore Boston Carlsbad Chicago Naples New York Philadelphia Portland
London Madrid Mexico City Singapore Sydney Tokyo Toronto Wiesbaden

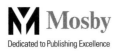

Mosby

Dedicated to Publishing Excellence

A Times Mirror
Company

Publisher: Don E. Ladig
Executive Editor: Martha Sasser
Associate Developmental Editor: Amy Dubin Christopher
Project Manager: John Rogers
Senior Production Editor: Helen Hudlin
Design Coordinator: Yael Kats
Series Design: Jeanne Wolfgeher
Manufacturing Supervisor: Theresa Fuchs
Editing and Production: Carlisle Publishers Services

Printed in the United States of America
Composition by Carlisle Communications, Ltd.
Printing/binding by Maple-Vail

Mosby–Year Book, Inc.
11830 Westline Industrial Drive
St. Louis, Missouri 63146

Library of Congress Cataloging-in-Publication Data

Contact lenses for pre- and post-surgery / edited by Michael G. Harris
  ; with 9 contributors.
     p.   cm. — (Mosby's optometric problem solving series)
  Includes bibliographical references and index.
  ISBN 0-8151-1400-1
  1. Contact lenses. 2. Eye—Surgery—Complications. I. Harris,
  [DNLM: 1. Contact Lenses. 2. Eye—Surgery. WW 355 C7617 1997]
  RE977.C6C5557 1997
  617.7'523—dc20
  DNLM/DLC
for Library of Congress   96–29286
                                         CIP

ISBN 0-8151-1400-1

97 98 99 00 / 9 8 7 6 5 4 3 2 1

Contributors

James V. Aquavella, MD
Clinical Professor of Ophthalmology
Director, Cornea Research Laboratory
University of Rochester
Rochester, New York

Edward Bennett, OD, FAAO
School of Optometry
University of Missouri—St. Louis
St. Louis, Missouri

Dennis Burger, OD, FAAO
Associate Clinical Professor
School of Optometry
University of California, Berkeley
Berkeley, California;
Senior Optometrist
Department of Optometry
Kaiser Permanente Medical Center
Oakland, California

Michael D. DePaolis, OD
Adjunct Professor of Optometry
Pennsylvania College of Optometry
Philadelphia, Pennsylvania

Lawrence A. Gans, MD
Eye Healthcare
Florissant, Missouri

Michael G. Harris, OD, JD, MS
Associate Dean
Clinical Professor
Chief, Contact Lens Clinic
School of Optometry
University of California, Berkeley
Berkeley, California

Anthony J. Phillips, MPhil, FBOA, HD, FBCO, FAAO, EAAO, EVCO, DCLP
Contact Lens Unit
Flinders Medical Centre
Women and Children's Hospital
Adelaide, South Australia

Joseph P. Shovlin, OD, FAAO
Clinical Associate
Northeastern Eye Institute
Scranton, Pennsylvania

Barry A. Weissman, OD, PhD, FAAO

Professor of Ophthalmology
Jules Stein Eye Institute and Department
of Ophthalmology
University of California, Los Angeles
School of Medicine
Los Angeles, California

Karla Zadnik, OD, PhD

Assistant Professor
Ohio State University
College of Optometry
Division of Epidemiology and
Biostatistics
School of Public Health
Ohio State University College
of Medicine
Columbus, Ohio

This book is dedicated to those who preceded me—my mentors:
Mort Sarver, Bob Mandell, Bob Lester, Irv Fatt, and Dick Hill.
It is also dedicated to those who will follow me—my students.

Preface

Contact lens specialists have long recognized the value of contact lenses in fitting pre- and post-ocular surgery patients. For these patients, contact lenses offer more than just the mere cosmetic benefit of not having to wear glasses. Contact lenses may be the only way these individuals can see and function in a modern society.

Because these patients' corneas may be affected by pre-existing disease, degeneration, or the after effects of surgery, contact lens fitting requires the utmost skill and dedication. This book is designed to provide practitioners and students with background information so that they can care for pre- and post-surgical contact lens patients.

In the first chapter, Bennett and Gans discuss the use of corneal topography in fitting pre- and post-surgical contact lens patients. In later chapters, Zadnik and Burger provide valuable insights on fitting contact lenses to keratoconic patients, Zadnik and Phillips offer expert advice on fitting therapeutic soft and rigid contact lenses to pre- and post-surgery patients, and Weissman discusses the application of contact lenses in the care and treatment in aphakia. Lastly Shovlin, DePaolis, and Aquavella discuss the emerging topic of fitting contact lenses to patients who have undergone refractive surgery.

The authors have done a marvelous job of providing valuable clinical insight into this specialized area of contact lens practice. In so doing, they provide contact lens practitioners with the foundation they need to be able to care for the unique problems of pre- and post-ocular surgery contact lens patients.

Michael G. Harris, OD, JD, MS

Acknowledgments

I thank the authors and the staffs of their practices and institutions for their time and effort in writing the chapters for this text. My special thanks to Brenda Marshall, who assisted in the preparation of this book.

My thanks also to Series Editor Dr. Richard London and to Martha Sasser, Amy Dubin, and the editorial production staff of Mosby–Year Book, Inc. for their assistance with this project.

Most importantly, I would like to thank my wife Dawn, my children, Matt, Dan, Ashley, and Lindsay, my parents, my friends, my colleagues, and my students for their love, friendship, and support.

Michael G. Harris, OD, JD, MS

Contents

1

Corneal Topography in Pre- and Post-Surgical Contact Lens Fitting

Edward S. Bennett
Lawrence Gans

Key Terms

corneal topography	penetrating	photorefractive
keratoconus	keratoplasty	keratectomy
	radial keratotomy	

The introduction of computerized videokeratographs (CVKs) has provided practitioners with the ability to comprehensively evaluate corneal curvature. Therefore the ability to both monitor and manage postoperative corneal conditions has been enhanced. Specifically, the contact lens management of these conditions is an important and ever-improving benefit of computerized videokeratographs.

Traditional Methods of Topography Evaluation

The keratometer has been the starting point for contact lens fitting because it is easy to use, relatively inexpensive, accurate, and its results are reproducible for normal corneal curvatures (40 to 46 D).[1] However, use of the keratometer assumes that the cornea is symmetric.[2,3] The keratometer determines four points around a circle measuring 2.8 to 4.0 mm, depending on the corneal power (i.e., for a 36 diopter [D] cornea, it measures a 4-mm zone; for a 50 D cornea, this measured zone decreases to 2.88 mm.)[1,4] Therefore the keratometer only evaluates the curvature of a few points of the central cornea. This extremely limited information is very disadvantageous when evaluating a patient with keratoconus, where the apex of the cone is almost always decentered, and in penetrating keratoplasty and refractive surgery cases in which the surface area of the affected region is typically much larger. In these cases (in addition to others involving irregular corneas), midperipheral and peripheral topography information is very important. Certainly it can be extremely difficult to achieve an adequate contact lens–to–fitting relationship on a patient having irregular astigmatism without the availability of more information to characterize corneal shape than that provided by the keratometer.

In the 1970s and 1980s several instruments were introduced to provide a qualitative analysis of corneal topography using a Placido disk image.[1,5] Examples of instruments that provided Polaroid photographic images of Placido rings projected onto the cornea were the Wesley-Jessen Photokeratoscope and the Corneascope (Kera Corporation). The former used seven rings, the latter nine (later expanded to twelve) rings for analysis. These instruments were important for providing the practitioner with more information about corneal topography and represented an important precursor to the CVK instruments available today. However, the accuracy was limited to 1 to 2 D and the quantitative analysis was time-consuming.

Computerized Videokeratograph Principles

The computerized videokeratograph uses the principle of projecting some form of light onto the cornea, where the light is modified and then photographed by a video camera. The computer software then captures, scans, and digitizes these reflections and the resulting data can be displayed in a wide variety of formats.[1,6] The most popular format is to use Placido disk reflectance in which a series of rings is projected onto the cornea with the reflected images detected by a video camera (Figure 1-1). The measured distances between the rings results in the derivation of curvature data. Among the most popular of the numerous formats used to show the data include a topographical map (Figure 1-2) and a numerical or tabular display (Figure 1-3). There is typically a lengthy list of available applications. Other technologies, in addition to Placido disk, that are present or forthcoming include laser holography, stereoasterography, and video optical-slit scanning.[6]

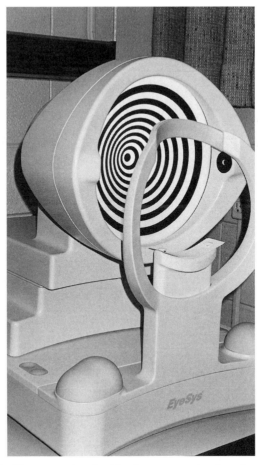

FIGURE 1-1 Computerized videokeratograph showing the Placido disk.

Computerized Videokeratograph Benefits and Applications

Corneal Curvature Analysis

CVK offers a reproducible and accurate method of measuring almost the entire corneal curvature, resulting in analysis of several thousand data points.[7-9] The algorithms for analysis of this data, however, assume that the cornea is spherical; therefore error in measurement increases with increases in astigmatism, asphericity, and irregularity of the corneal surface.[10-12] Nevertheless, CVK instruments can analyze a large amount of information and show this information in a variety of useful formats. The most common and beneficial format is the color map (see Plates 2 to 4). Originally developed in 1987,[13] the

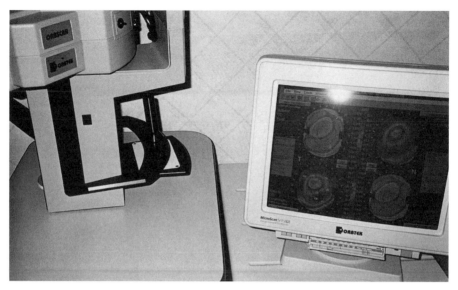

FIGURE 1-2 Computerized videokeratograph with accompanying color map.

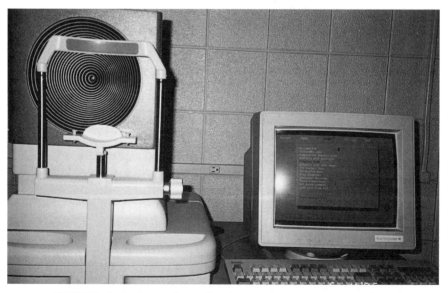

FIGURE 1-3 List of applications of a computerized videokeratograph.

color map has since been expanded and improved.[14,15] It was derived using an axial (sagittal) radius of curvature. The map offers the examiner instant recognition of the topography of almost the entire cornea. It provides information that can be used at baseline and to monitor changes over time caused by keratoconus, refractive surgery, or some other corneal condition. Likewise the color map can be used to assist in contact lens selection and to evaluate the effect of contact lens wear over time on corneal topography. One practical benefit of the color map is that patients can readily understand their topography as the practitioner explains that cooler colors such as blue represent a less curved or flatter corneal contour while hotter colors such as red represent a more curved or steeper contour. Many practices provide a copy of the map for their patients to take home. This not only enhances patient satisfaction but also encourages better cooperation via increased knowledge. Typically, not only can color maps and other applications be printed on high-quality color laser printers, but, with the appropriate software, they can be developed into 35mm slides.

In addition to sagittal color maps, data from CVKs can also be presented tangentially. Tangential or instantaneous curvature plots are derived by placing a tangent to each of the data points on the CVK and determining the radius from the tangent rather than from the sagittal plane.[6,16] They are not axis dependent and reads as though the CVK was realigned for every point on the cornea. Therefore the tangential radius of curvature can provide a more accurate shape analysis for peripheral corneal powers and is beneficial for patients with keratoconus, contact lenses, and irregular and postsurgical corneas.

Multiple color maps can be used to show changes or differences in topography. Most CVK software programs have the ability to produce a difference map, which compares a current color map with an earlier map to give an indication of topography changes over time. The difference map represents an arithmetic subtraction of one topography map from another. Likewise, many programs have the ability to show as many as four color maps simultaneously, which is very beneficial in viewing topography changes over time, particularly in postsurgical cases.

Numerical values for corneal curvature data points are also demonstrated in a variety of formats. One format is a color-coded, numerical representation in which the radius of curvature values is shown in a radial pattern along meridians, which are at designated degree separations (i.e., 15°). Many systems show the data in a tabular format in which the diopters, radius of curvature in millimeters, and distance from the center point for each of the calculated data points are shown in columns. Keratometric-like data are also common to these systems. Data from the central 3 mm of the cornea can be averaged, and simulated keratometric readings provided. These keratometric values are typically based on averaging a much larger number of data points than are available in conventional keratometry. In addition, average values from the midperiphery and periphery of the cornea are often provided.

Other applications common to many of the CVK instruments include a profile map, an eye image map, and pupil simulation. A profile map plots diopter changes over the corneal surface. A reproduction of the original video image of the patient's eye complete with Placido rings and a simulated pupil zone is another option. The use of special image subtraction and enhancement techniques to locate the patient's pupil is very beneficial in determining centration during refractive surgery.[1]

Contact Lens Fitting

A logical development of CVK is application in contact lens fitting where many—and ever-increasing—benefits are present. By providing a qualitative and quantitative evaluation of a much larger corneal area than that provided by keratometry, CVK provides a better estimate of the base-curve fitting relationship.[6,17,18] In particular, the color map can assist in locating and determining the curvature of the corneal apex and can also indicate the approximate range of change of curvature of the cornea.[16]

The introduction of newer, more accurate, and comprehensive contact lens software packages has allowed the practitioner to obtain a large amount of corneal information and then recommend lens design information based on corneal topography, viewing the effect on a simulated fluorescein pattern. The latter is a very useful application of CVK because a simulated fluorescein pattern can be viewed before diagnostic lens application. The proximity of the posterior lens surface to the anterior surface of the cornea and the thickness of the layer of tear fluid in between can be viewed in various shades of green. Any lens parameter can be changed and the resultant fluorescein pattern can be recalculated and displayed along with the patient's corneal topography[18,19] (Plate 1).

This allows lens fitting with a pre-evaluation of the actual lens base curve-to-cornea relationship via the tear lens thickness, rather than a numerical estimate provided by keratometry.[19] This can potentially reduce patient chair time and simplify the fitting process by providing more comprehensive and accurate fitting information before diagnostic lens application.

There have been reports of 90% or more patients having a similar fluorescein pattern with their actual lens as that simulated with CVK contact lens software.[20,21] When differences do exist, they may be attributed to software limitations such as lack of simulated lens movement, flexure and lid position and tension, in addition to the aforementioned inaccuracies of currently available topography instrument data in the corneal periphery.[10,19] However, the contact lens software programs continue to improve; for example, the Pro-Fit program (EyeSys) incorporates decentration and tilt functions. Although almost all software programs provide simulated fluorescein pattern and recommended computer-assisted lens design application based on a particular algorithm, there are some differences between programs. These programs are listed in Table 1-1.[22]

CLINICAL PEARL

CVK can potentially reduce patient chair time and simplify the fitting process by providing more comprehensive and accurate fitting information before diagnostic lens application.

It is important to mention that CVK instruments do not replace diagnostic fitting, especially in patients with irregular corneas. They do, however, greatly assist in determining the initial diagnostic lenses and should reduce the number of lenses necessary to achieve a desirable lens-to-cornea fitting relationship. The software programs typically have a recommended design philosophy, which should result in an alignment or near alignment–simulated fluorescein pattern. The practitioner can also typically custom design lenses as well.

The benefits of contact lens software on production of higher quality rigid gas-permeable (RGP) lenses and office efficiency appears to be quite good. Several manufacturers are interfacing their CNC computer-driving lathes with CVK software programs so that, via modem, the practitioner can send topography information and lens parameters directly to the manufacturer.

Keratoconus

One of the most important applications of CVK instrumentation is the diagnosis, monitoring, and contact lens or surgical management of keratoconus. There have been many documented cases of subclinical keratoconus in which the keratometry and slit lamp findings were not indicative of keratoconus, but a decentered steep conical area, characteristic of early keratoconus, was diagnosed with CVK.[23-25] Keratoconus can be diagnosed earlier in patients and management—typically with RGP contact lenses—can result in an immediate improvement in

TABLE 1-1

Corneal Topography Instruments Contact Lens Software

Contact Lens Fitting	Alcon Surgical	Alliance Medical Mktg	EyeSys Technologies	Humphrey Instruments	Kera Metrics	Technomed GMBH	Tomey Technology	Topcon America Corp
Model	EH-290	Keratron Analyzer	2000	Mastervue 910/920	KM-CLAS-1000	CSCAN	TMS-2	CM-1000
Module, included/available cost	Avail		Incl	$1500		Incl		Avail
Fitting strategies (AC, AL, AS)*	AC	AC, AL, AS		AC, AL, AS	AS		AC, AL, AS	AS
Other			User defined	Keratometric, topographic	Optical subtraction	SRM-method/top test		
Simulated fluorescein	•	•	•	•			•	•
Contact lens tilt								
Automatic	•	•	•					
Manual						•	•	•
Both		•		•				
Sagittal tear-film plots	•	•	•				•	
Lens positioning adjustments		•	•				•	
Print contact lens parameters	•	•	•	•		•	•	•

*AC = apical clearance; AL = alignment; AS = aspheric.
From *Buyer's Guide to Corneal Topography*, *EyeCare Technol* 5(4):24-25, 1995.

8

visual acuity. In addition, the use of CVK can assist the practitioner in determining the region and size of the conical area.

CLINICAL PEARL

There have been many documented cases of subclinical keratoconus in which the keratometry and slit lamp findings were not indicative of keratoconus, but a decentered steep conical area, characteristic of early keratoconus, was diagnosed with CVK.

Several characteristic features diagnostic of keratoconus are determined via CVK. These include:
- Central corneal power > 47 D
- Difference of ≥ 3 D between points 3 mm above center to 3 mm below center
- Asymmetry between central corneal power of fellow eyes in excess of 1 D

The use of serial topographic examinations will help in monitoring the progression of keratoconus while differentiating it from other conditions such as corneal warpage syndrome or a lid attachment lens-to-cornea fitting relationship. A superior decentering rigid contact lens can induce a pseudo-keratoconic corneal topographical pattern in which the superior cornea flattens in curvature while the inferior cornea steepens.[6,27] This condition can be diagnosed by observing the fitting relationship and noting that, if the lenses are removed, the inferior cornea quickly flattens toward baseline (Figure 1-4).

CVK is very beneficial for screening keratoconus in refractive surgical candidates as this pre-existing pathology would be a contraindication for surgery (Plate 2). Studies have resulted in approximately 5% to 7% of potential refractive surgery candidates being diagnosed as having subclinical keratoconus.[28,29] This high percentage may be indicative of these patients' dissatisfaction with their current mode of correction. The color map can provide an effective visual aid to help the patient understand why refractive surgery is not advisable.

CLINICAL PEARL

CVK is very beneficial for screening keratoconus in refractive surgical candidates as this pre-existing pathology would be a contraindication for surgery.

Contact lens fitting for keratoconus can be greatly enhanced with CVK. The color map provides information about the size, location,

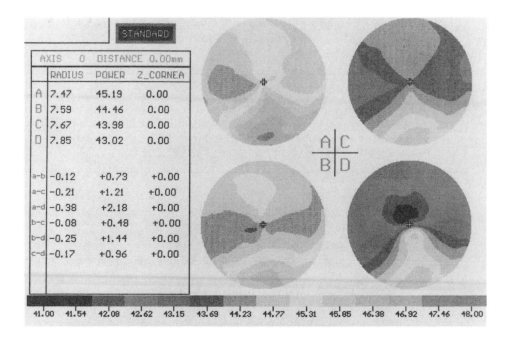

AXIS	0	DISTANCE	0.00mm
	RADIUS	POWER	Z_CORNEA
A	7.47	45.19	0.00
B	7.59	44.46	0.00
C	7.67	43.98	0.00
D	7.85	43.02	0.00
a-b	-0.12	+0.73	+0.00
a-c	-0.21	+1.21	+0.00
a-d	-0.38	+2.18	+0.00
b-c	-0.08	+0.48	+0.00
b-d	-0.25	+1.44	+0.00
c-d	-0.17	+0.96	+0.00

41.00 41.54 42.08 42.62 43.15 43.69 44.23 44.77 45.31 45.85 46.38 46.92 47.46 48.00

FIGURE 1-4 Case of pseudo-keratoconus in which the color map immediately after lens removal appears to show an inferior keratoconic-like pattern *(A)*, However, 45 minutes after removal *(B)*, 1½ hours after removal *(C)*, and 2½ hours after removal *(D)*, the inferior cornea gradually flattens toward baseline as an example of a lid attachment RGP-fitting relationship.

and curvature of the apex of the cone. As the apex is almost always decentered and a rigid contact lens tends to gravitate to the steepest region of the cornea, the color map will assist in determining if a larger diameter and/or aspheric lens design may be needed to provide centration in these cases. Likewise, although the contact lens software programs are more prone to error with irregular astigmatism, the simulated fluorescein and recommended lens parameters can provide an important starting point for diagnostic fitting. I tend to use the flatter simulated keratometry value as a starting point for diagnostic fitting. If central bearing is present, I select gradually steeper base curve radii until apical clearance is first achieved; then, the previous lens that exhibited mild apical bearing is selected. Likewise, contact lens software typically provides edge lift values. It is important to have a greater edge lift design (i.e., flatter, wide peripheral curve) than with conventional lens designs to minimize adherence (Figure 1-5). In fact, values of .25 mm to .4 mm as compared to the customary .08 mm to .12 mm have been recommended.[6]

My fitting philosophy is summarized in Box 1-1.

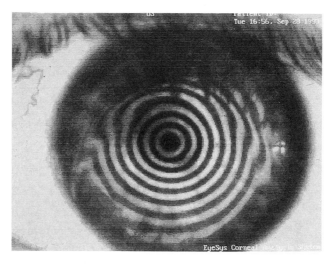

FIGURE 1-5 Imprint or adherence ring of a keratoconic patient immediately after removal of an adherent RGP lens.

═══ Box 1-1   Recommended Keratoconus-Fitting Guidelines

- Use computerized videokeratography to assist in determining the location, size, and curvature of the apex of the cone.
- Select a base curve equal to the flatter simulated keratometry as a starting point. If apical bearing is present, gradually steepen the base curve radius until apical clearance is present; then select the previous lens.
- Always use diagnostic lenses and evaluate the fluorescein pattern with the assistance of a yellow filter over the observation system. If possible, use a Burton lamp for fluorescein pattern observation to provide a greater field of view.
- Select an optical zone diameter similar to the base curve radius (in millimeters).
- The use of anywhere from two to four peripheral curves is important to provide an adequate fitting relationship. A higher edge lift design is necessary to allow good tear exchange and to minimize adherence. The contact lens software program can assist in providing edge lift values in the .25 to .40 mm range. Typically, the peripheral curve radius will be at least 12 mm, having a width equal to a minimum of .3 mm to .4 mm.

The following case will demonstrate how CVK is beneficial in achieving a successful lens-to-cornea fitting relationship.

Case One: Keratoconus

Patient AA complained of blurred vision and gradual reduction in comfort with her present RGP lenses. Data for lenses were verified as the following:

	OD	OS
Base Curve Radius	7.30mm	7.30mm
Overall Diameter	8.80mm	8.80mm
Optical Zone Diameter	7.40mm	7.40mm
Power	−4.00 D	−5.25 D

Slit lamp evaluation revealed excessive movement with blink, inferior decentration, and central bearing with fluorescein instillation. Observation of her corneal topography data revealed that keratoconus in the left eye was more progressive than in the right eye, having a steepest curvature of 72.62 vs. 60.26 D OD and simulated keratometry readings of OD: 48.49 @ 008, 54.34 @ 098 and OS: 57.98 @ 159, 62.84 @ 069 (Figure 1-6).

The patient was fitted initially on the flatter simulated K reading OU. As each lens exhibited apical clearance, three-point touch was ultimately established with a base curve radius of 7.10 mm OD, and 6.80 mm OS. As the affected area was relatively small and only slightly decentered inferiorly, good centration was obtained. The final lens design included the following lens parameters:

	OD	OS
Lens Material	Fluoroperm	30 OU
Base Curve Radius	7.10 mm	6.80 mm
Overall Diameter	8.60 mm	8.60 mm
Optical Zone Diameter	7.20 mm	7.00 mm
Power	−6.00 D	−7.25 D
Secondary Curve Radius/Width	9.00/.3 mm	8.00/.2 mm
Intermediate Curve Radius/Width		9.6/.3 mm
Peripheral Curve Radius/Width	12.00/.4 mm	12.00/.3 mm
	Plus lenticular OU	

Penetrating Keratoplasty (PK)

CVK provides numerous benefits for post-penetrating keratoplasty patients, including initial evaluation, monitoring of topography changes, and contact lens fitting. Conventional keratometry is often precluded in post-penetrating keratoplasty evaluation as these patient's corneas have highly variable curvatures, both centrally and at

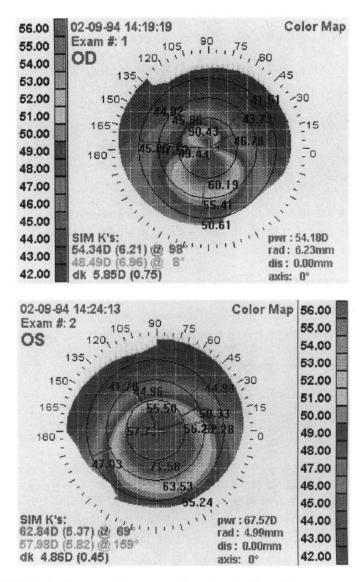

FIGURE 1-6 Topography maps of patient in Case One.

the wound margin.[30] In the post-penetrating keratoplasty cornea, the apical zone may not be centrally located; therefore, conventional keratometry may have an even higher error rate.[31] Variability in topography readings—even with the same observer[31]—can be observed with CVK on a post-penetrating keratoplasty cornea because, in part, of the difficulty in visualizing the peripheral focusing aids and because of increased error with irregular corneal surfaces. Nevertheless, CVK provides much more quantitiative analysis than keratometry or photokeratoscopy, even with high cylindrical aberrations.[30,32] It is also very helpful in determining what type of graft is present (i.e., conventional, sunken, proud, tilted, or displaced). Likewise, CVK is important in the monitoring of the post-PK cornea until stabilization has been achieved.

CVK can assist in contact lens design and fitting of post-PK patients. Because of the irregularity of the cornea in such patients, an RGP lens is indicated. As with other types of corneas, an RGP lens will always attempt to position over the area of greatest steepening.[16,33] CVK can both identify this area, and, also, with the use of simulated fluorescein pattern software, show the lens-to-cornea fitting relationship in this region. The use of the decentration and tilt functions, if present, are very beneficial in these cases.

CLINICAL PEARL

CVK can both identify this area, and, also, with the use of simulated fluorescein pattern software, show the lens-to-cornea fitting relationship in this region.

As with other patients with irregular corneas, diagnostic fitting is imperative in post-penetrating keratoplasty. CVK, however, has been found to be a much better predictor than keratometry of the ultimate base curve radius selected via diagnostic fitting.[31,32] Lopatynsky et al.[31] used CVK to fit 19 post-PK eyes with RGP lenses. They used the curvature value at 1.5 mm superior to center to determine the initial base curve radius. A superior-central position with good lens movement was their goal. The results of this study determined that there was no statistically significant difference between the base curve of the initially dispensed lens and the base curve of the lens worn after 3 months although modifications in the lens fit were required in 9 of 19 patients. However, a significant difference existed between the base curve radius initially recommended via CVK and that which would have been recommended by conventional keratometry, the latter almost always being flatter in curvature.

Typically, a large diameter lens is fit over the sutures in post-PK patients. As with keratoconus, the use of a high edge lift design ensures peripheral clearance and minimizes adherence. A value of .15 mm has been recommended, and this or a similar value can be input into the contact lens software and the resulting simulated fluorescein pattern will show if a lesser or greater peripheral clearance is indicated.[19] Both aspheric and multicurve spherical designs have achieved success in post-PK corneas, particularly when CVK has assisted in the design.[19,33,34]

CVK can also assist in monitoring changes in corneal topography with contact lens wear. It has been found that RGP lenses act as a splint or mold and will decrease corneal astigmatism and increase surface regularity.[32,35] The amount of astigmatism reduction can be as much as 3 D in early postoperative cases (i.e., 3 to 6 months).[35] However, a rigid lens that is decentered can cause greater surface irregularity. It has been recommended that performing either relaxing incisions or wedge resections in these cases may result in an improved lens-to-cornea fitting relationship by achieving greater symmetry around the visual axis of the corneal graft.[33]

Refractive Surgery

There are several benefits to using CVK for evaluating potential refractive surgery candidates and for postsurgical purposes. As discussed previously, CVK can rule out pre-existing pathology such as keratoconus, which, in many cases, would not be detected with keratometry. Likewise, decentration of refractive corneal procedures can result in blurred images, glare, ghost images, or poor visual acuity.[36,37] It has been determined that the best optical reference for refractive surgical procedures is the pupil center and not necessarily the visual axis. With the introduction of new pupil recognition software, CVK can now be used to determine if corneal refractive procedures have been properly centered.[38]

Another benefit of CVK is monitoring the cornea's healing response after refractive surgery. The use of serial maps to observe changes over time is particularly beneficial. Serial maps are beneficial for contact lens fitting as well because the practitioner can determine when corneal stability has occurred and then use the corneal topography data to assist in the lens design process and monitor the effect of the lens on corneal topography over time.

CLINICAL PEARL

The use of serial maps to observe changes over time is particularly beneficial.

Radial Keratotomy (RK)

The corneal topographical changes that typically accompany radial keratotomy include central corneal flattening, which varies in size, shape, and location.[39,40] The cornea has a so-called "knee" or area of rapid steepening in the midperiphery and a normal or slightly steeper periphery. Typically, the area of flattening or posterior displacement of corneal topography averages about 6 mm, whereas the anterior displacement or steepening of the midperipheral to peripheral cornea is located in the 6 mm to 11 mm area.[41] Through use of such topographical software formats as viewing serial and difference maps, the topographical changes induced by radial keratotomy can be monitored. One such format is the Standard Topographical Analysis for Refractive Surgery (STARS) Display (EyeSys), which provides a retrospective view of the cornea and helps analyze surgical results while tracking the healing process. This display actually shows five maps simultaneously: the preoperative, postoperative, and follow-up maps at the top, and the surgical change (difference between maps 1 and 2) and healing change difference maps at the bottom (difference between maps 2 and 3).

Once the cornea has stabilized, CVK is beneficial in the contact lens fitting process. The corneal topography often dictates a reverse curve lens design to provide good midperipheral alignment when the secondary curve is actually steeper than the base curve. The topographical maps help the practitioner determine if such a design is indicated and, if so, how much steeper the secondary curve should be from the base curve radius (i.e., typically it can be anywhere from 1 to 5 D steeper). Usually a large diameter lens (i.e., 9.5 mm to 10.5 mm) is fit either slightly steeper than the postoperative flat simulated keratometry value or slightly flatter than the preoperative simulated keratometry value. Slight apical clearance with midperipheral alignment is desirable. Radial keratotomy lens design and fitting are discussed in greater length in Chapter 6. A representative case is presented below.

Case Two: Radial Keratotomy

Patient SH had radial keratotomy and entered our clinic for a contact lens fitting. Her corneal topography was stable and her manifest refraction and simulated keratometer readings were as follows:

Manifest Refraction	Simulated Keratometry Readings
OD: P1 − 1.75 × 026 20/20	OD: 38.88/40.27
OS: −1.25 − 0.50 × 180 20/20	OS: 39.38/40.08

Her corneal topography exhibited characteristic central flattening and midperipheral steepening (Plate 3). She was fit with the Menicon Plateau lens, which is typically fit 1 D steeper than the postoperative flat keratometry reading and is available in reverse curves, which are either 2 D, 3 D, or 4 D steeper than the base curve. After diagnostic fitting, a steeper base curve radius than predicted OU (i.e., 8.22 mm) was found to provide good centration and the 2 D reverse curve resulted in optimum midperipheral alignment. The following lenses were ordered and resulted in a successful fit:

	OU
Lens Material/Design	Menicon Plateau
Base Curve Radius	8.22mm
Overall Diameter	10.0mm
Reverse Curve	2 D Steep

Photorefractive Keratectomy (PRK)

The topography of corneas that have experienced excimer laser photorefractive keratectomy (PRK) typically differs greatly from corneas altered by radial keratotomy. Usually, some mild central—but often uniform—flattening is observed in over 95% of the cases, but it is limited to the 5 mm to 6 mm ablated zone; corneal topography is essentially unchanged outside of the ablated zone.[42,43] This is a type I response. In a type II response, observed in 1% to 3% of patients, excessive central flattening is observed. About 1% to 3% of patients manifest a type III response in which corneal haze and regression of the refractive effect occur.[42,44] Central corneal flattening is limited and, in fact, the cornea is typically steepened in the region of the haze.[45] One potential complication of PRK is the so-called "central island," in which the central cornea has steepened more than 1.50 D and the affected region is greater than 1.5 mm in diameter[42,46] (Plate 4). The central island may be caused by such factors as hydration of the stroma following epithelial debridement or laser beam inhomogeneity. CVK is an excellent means of being able to monitor the topography changes of the central island over time since the phenomenon typically resolves over a 3-month period.

CVK can provide useful preoperative information about the location of the ablation zone, the amount of spherocylindrical aberration, and, if indicated, can monitor change after discontinuation of contact lens wear before surgery. Once stability has been achieved after surgery, contact lens fitting is typically more straightforward than post-RK fitting. Although a PRK-fitting software program has not been developed, use of color maps to observe the topography change and use of simulated fluorescein patterns to estimate the optimum lens design information are beneficial aids. With the exception of type II and type III responders, who exhibit more radical topographic changes and require a longer time period for stability, PRK patients are much easier to fit than post-RK patients because the central 5 to 6 mm of the cornea has been somewhat flattened but the midperiphery and periphery are unaltered. These patients can be fit with either a soft or RGP lens material; the latter has the benefit of being fit earlier in the process while the cornea is still healing as a result of material oxygen permeability and molding benefits. A reverse curve design is almost always unnecessary and either a conventional spherical or aspheric lens design will be successful.[47,48]

Summary

Use of computerized videokeratography is a valuable tool for the management of the patient with an irregular cornea. Applications such as diagnosis of keratoconus, comprehensive quantiative analysis of pre- and postsurgical corneal topography, and monitoring of corneal change over time are important applications of this new technology. However, contact lens applications are especially beneficial in the management of these patients, and the introduction of newer and more updated contact lens software should result in an even more efficient and successful fitting process.

References

1. Koch DD, Haft EA: Introduction to corneal topography. In Sanders DR, Koch DD: *An atlas of corneal topography,* Thorofare, NJ, 1993, Slack, Inc, 1-32.
2. Dabezies OJ, Holladay J: Measurement of corneal curvature: keratometer (ophthalmometer). In Dabezies OJ, Farris L, Lemp M, eds: *Contact lenses: the CLAO guide to basic science and clinical practice,* Orlando, 1984, Grune & Stratton, 17.1-17.29.
3. Clark BAJ: Mean topography of normal corneas, *Aust J Optom* 57:107-114, 1974.
4. Binder PS: Videokeratography, *CLAO J* 21(2):133-143, 1995.
5. Rowsey JJ, Reynolds AE, Brown R: Corneal topography, *Arch Ophthalmol* 99:1093-1100, 1981.
6. Lebow KA, Schnider CM: Corneal topography and contact lens fitting, *Optom Today* Jan-Feb:55-68, 1996.
7. Dindeldein SA, Klyce SD: Topography of normal corneas, *Arch Ophthalmol* 107:512-518, 1989.
8. Hannush SB, Crawford SL, Waring GO, et al: Accuracy and precision of keratometry, photokeratoscopy, and corneal modeling on calibrated steel balls, *Arch Ophthalmol* 107:1235-1239, 1989.
9. Hannush SB, Crawford SL, Waring GO, et al: Reproducibility of normal corneal power measurements with a keratometer, photokeratoscopy, and Video Imaging System, *Arch Ophthalmol* 108:539-544, 1990.
10. Roberts C: Characteristics of the inherent error in a spherically-biased corneal topography system in mapping a radially aspheric surface, *J Refract Corneal Surg* 10:103-116, 1994.
11. Antalis JJ, Lembach RG, Carney LG: A comparison of the TMS-a and the Corneal Analysis System for the evaluation of abnormal corneas, *CLAO J* 19:58-63, 1993.
12. Nguyen NN, Applegate RA: Measurement accuracy of corneal videokeratographic (VK) systems using aspheric and simulated PRK surfaces, *Invest Ophthalmol Vis Sci* (suppl):1217, 1993.
13. Maguire L, Singer D, Klyce SD: Graphic presentation of computer-analyzed keratoscope photographs, *Arch Ophthalmol* 105:223-230, 1987.
14. Dingeldein S, Klyce S: Imaging the cornea, *Cornea* 7:170-182, 1988.

15. Wilson S, Klyce S, Husseini Z: Standardized color-coded maps for corneal topography, *Ophthalmology* 100:1723-1727, 1993.
16. Soper B: Pro-fit fitting manual, Houston, TX, 1995, EyeSys Technologies.
17. Wasserman D, Itzkowitz J, Kamenas T, Asbell PA: Corneal topographic data: its use in fitting aspheric contact lenses, *CLAO J* 18(2):83-85, 1992.
18. Stevenson RWW, Corbett MD, O'Brart PS, Rosen ES: Corneal topography in contact lens practice, *Eur J Implant Ref Surg* 7:305-317, 1995.
19. Szczotka LB, Reinhart W: Computerized videokeratoscopy contact lens software for RGP fitting in a bilateral postkeratoplasty patient: a clinical case report, *CLAO J* 21(1):52-56, 1995.
20. Dubow B: Corneal topography and RGP fitting in a managed care world, *Eyecare Technol* Jan:61-63, 1996.
21. Soper B, Shovlin J, Bennett ES: A topography-based RGP contact lens fitting algorithm, *Austral Optom (AO)* April:7-10, 1996.
22. Buyer's guide to corneal topography, *Eyecare Technol* 5(4):24-25, 1995.
23. Maeda N, Klyce SD: Videokeratography in contact lens practice, *Int Contact Lens Clin* 21(9 & 10):163-168, 1994.
24. Maguire LJ, Bourne WM: Corneal topography of early keratoconus, *Am J Ophthalmol* 108:107-112, 1989.
25. Morrow G, Stein RM: Evaluation of corneal topography: past, present and furure trends, *Can J Ophthalmol* 27(5):213-224, 1992.
26. Rabinowitz YS, McDonnell PJ: Computer-assisted corneal topography in keratoconus, *Refract Corneal Surg* 5:400-408, 1989.
27. Buscemi P: Corneal topography: a quantum leap in contact lens design, *Optom Today* Sept:45-46, 1995.
28. Wilson SD, Klyce SD: Screening for corneal topographic abnormalities before refractive surgery, *Ophthalmology* 101:147-152, 1994.
29. Nesburn AB, Bahri S, Berlin M, et al: Computer-Assisted Corneal Topography (CACT) to detect mild keratoconus in candidates for photorefractive keratectomy, *Invest Ophthalmol Vis Sci* 33/4 (suppl):995, 1992.
30. Manabe R, Matsuda M, Suda T: Photokeratoscopy in fitting contact lenses after penetrating keratoscopy, *Br J Ophthalmol* 70:55-59, 1986.
31. Lopatynsky M, Cohen EJ, Leavitt KG, Laibson PR: Corneal topography for rigid gas permeable lens fitting after penetrating keratoplasty, *CLAO J* 19(1):41-44, 1993.
32. Sperber LTD, Lopatynsky MO, Cohen EJ: Corneal topography in contact lens wearers following penetrating keratoplasty, *CLAO J* 21(3):183-189, 1995.
33. Koffler BH, Clements LD, Litteral GL, Smith VM: A new contact lens design for post-keratoplasty patients, *CLAO J* 20(3):170-175, 1994.
34. Weiner BM, Nirankari VS: A new biaspheric contact lens for severe astigmatism following penetrating keratoplasty, *CLAO J* 18(1):29-33, 1992.
35. Wilson SE, Friedman RS, Klyce SD: Contact lens manipulation of corneal topography after penetrating keratoplasty: a preliminary study, *CLAO J* 18(3):177-182, 1992.
36. Uozato H, Guyton DL: Centering corneal surgical procedures, *Am J Ophthalmol* 103:264-275, 1987.
37. Walsh PM, Guyton DL: Comparison of two methods of marking the visual axis on the cornea during radial keratotomy, *Am J Ophthalmol* 97:660, 1984.
38. Sanders DR: Evaluating refractive surgical or laser procedures. In Sanders DR, Koch DD: *An atlas of corneal topography*, Thorofare, NJ, 1993, Slack, Inc, 85-92.
39. McDonnell PJ, Garbus J: Corneal topographic changes after radial keratotomy, *Ophthalmology* 96(1):45-49, 1989.
40. Rowsey JJ, Balyeat HD, Monlux R, et al: Prospective evaluation of radial keratotomy: photokeratoscope corneal topography, *Ophthalmology* 95:322-334, 1988.
41. Bogan SJ, Maloney RK, Drews CD, Waring GO: Computer-assisted videokeratography of corneal topography after radial keratotomy, *Arch Ophthalmol* 109:834-841, 1991.

42. Karpecki PM, Smith JM, Durrie DS: What you can do to improve PRK outcomes, *Rev Optom* 133(3):127-133, 1996.

43. Johnson DD: Excimer PRK: ready for takeoff, *Rev Optom* 132(1):80-82, 1995.

44. Durrie DS, Lesher MP, Cavanaugh TB: Classification of variable clinical response after myopic photorefractive keratectomy. In *Medical cornea-corneal and refractive surgery*, Amsterdam/New York, 1994, Kugler Publications, 127-140.

45. Grimm B, Waring GO, Ibrahim O: Regional variation in corneal topography and wound healing following photorefractive keratectomy *J Refract Surg* 11:348-355, 1995.

46. DePaolis MD, Aquavella J: When is additional surgery necessary? *Contact Lens Spectrum* 10(3):45, 1995.

47. McLaughlin R: Follow the fluctuating fit post-PRK, *Contact Lens Spectrum* 10(6):44, 1995.

48. Schipper I, Businger U, Pfarrer R: Fitting contact lenses after excimer laser photorefractive keratectomy for myopia, *CLAO J* 21(4):281-283, 1995.

C H A P T E R

2

Keratoconus

Dennis Burger
Karla Zadnik

Key Terms

keratoconus	contact lenses	corneal diseases
cornea	corneal	visual acuity
astigmatism	transplantation	

Keratoconus is a noninflammatory, self-limiting ectasia of the axial portion of the cornea[1] characterized by progressive thinning and steepening of the central cornea. As the cornea steepens and thins, the patient experiences a decrease in vision that can be mild or severe depending on the amount of corneal tissue affected. Typically, vision loss can be corrected early by spectacles; later, irregular astigmatism requires correction with rigid contact lenses.[2] Contact lenses provide a uniform refracting surface and therefore improve vision.

When keratoconus is first diagnosed, the patient should be informed of the following:

1. Contact lenses will eventually be necessary
2. About 20% of patients eventually need corneal surgery[3,4]
3. The cornea may scar even if contact lenses are worn
4. Prognosis is unpredictable and progression is variable
5. Annual or more frequent eye examinations are indicated
6. The disease does not cause blindness, but may compromise quality of life, although keratoconus patients can usually still drive and read

The incidence of keratoconus in the general population is .15% to .6%.[5-9] Onset of keratoconus occurs during the teenage years—mean age of onset is 16 years[7,10]—but onset has occurred in patients as young as 6 years old.[1,11] Keratoconus rarely develops after age 30.[10] Keratoconus shows no gender predilection and is bilateral in 90% of cases.[5,8,12] In general, the disease develops asymmetrically; diagnosis of the disease in the second eye lags about 5 years behind diagnosis in the first.[6] The disease process is active for about 5 to 7 years,[1,6,8,9] and then may be stable for many years. During the active stage, change may be rapid; contact lenses may have to be refit as often as every 3 to 4 months. Pregnancy may cause the disease process to become active.[7]

Etiology

The proposed etiologies of keratoconus include corneal tissue changes, heredity, atopic disease, systemic disorders, and rigid contact lens wear.

Corneal tissue change has long been proposed as a cause of keratoconus; debate has focused on whether the primary site is the stroma or the epithelium and its basement membrane. Teng[13] originally proposed the epithelium as the primary site of abnormal tissue because the earliest histopathological change occurs there. Many researchers now believe that the primary site is the stroma and that tissue change occurs because of destruction of stromal tissue by collagenase.[14-16]

The role of heredity as a possible cause of keratoconus has been studied.[17,18] Keratoconus may be inherited as a dominant or recessive trait.[6,9] Hammerstein[18] found that in families in which one member had keratoconus, the incidence of keratoconus in other family members was 8%. Rabinowitz et al[17] showed a high prevalence of nonkeratoconic corneal topographical abnormalities among family members of keratoconus patients.

Atopic disease (e.g., hay fever, atopic dermatitis, or asthma) also has been suggested as an etiological component of keratoconus.[19] Rahi et al[19] found atopic disease in 35% of keratoconus patients, compared with 12% of normal patients. The known immunological disturbance associated with atopic disease—raised serum levels of immunoglobulin E—was present in 47% to 52% of keratoconus patients.[19,20] Ridley's[10] eye-rubbing theory may be related to this observation; Ridley noted that keratoconus patients are chronic eye rubbers, and he theorized that rubbing indents the cornea, increases intraocular pressure, and may make the cornea yield at its weakest point, the center.[9,21,22] However, patients with atopic disease may rub their eyes because of the atopic condition and the itching it causes.[20]

Many systemic conditions have been linked to keratoconus. Bennett[1] listed these conditions as Down syndrome, Ehlers-Danlos syndrome (a connective tissue disorder in which the skin is loosely attached to the bones), Rieger's syndrome (posterior embryotoxon), Crouzon's syndrome (craniofacial dysostosis), and Marfan's syndrome.

A final proposed cause of keratoconus is rigid contact lens wear. It has been theorized that long-term wear of rigid contact lenses may trigger keratoconus in patients predisposed to the disease.[22-26] Studies were retrospective and showed no direct cause and effect between wearing rigid contact lenses and the development of keratoconus. Most research documented PMMA lens wear; no study of which we are aware has found any association between keratoconus and gas-permeable rigid or soft contact lens wear. Macsai et al[27] retrospectively reviewed keratoconus patients at the University of Iowa to determine whether keratoconus preceded rigid lens wear or vice versa. Results of the study showed that patients who wore rigid contact lenses before diagnosis of keratoconus had less severe disease (i.e., flatter corneas) and were older when diagnosed.

To date, no single, clear-cut cause of keratoconus has been found. The various proposed causes may interact: atopic disease may interact with rigid contact lens wear, ocular trauma may interact with decreased ocular rigidity, or as Mandell[28] theorized, keratoconus might be part of an as yet unidentified systemic syndrome.

Diagnosis

Although identifying moderate or advanced keratoconus is fairly easy, diagnosing the disease in its early stages is often difficult. An accurate case history is vital. Often keratoconus patients have had several spectacle prescriptions in a short period, and none has provided satisfactory vision correction. Keratoconus patients often report monocular diplopia or polyopia and complain of distortion at both distant and near vision. Halos around lights and photophobia may be reported.

Visual and refractive clues may be present. The early keratoconus patient may have reduced visual acuity in one eye because of the disease's asymmetry. This sign is often associated with oblique astigmatism. In early keratoconus the patient may become less myopic 6 months into the disease process as astigmatism increases. The −2.00 D myopic patient who develops a refractive error of −1.50 = −1.00 ax 155 may be developing keratoconus.

Many objective signs are present in keratoconus. Retinoscopy shows a scissoring reflex.[6,7,29] Direct ophthalmoscopy may show a shadow. If the pupil is dilated and a +6.00 D lens is in the ophthalmoscopic system, the cone may resemble an oil or honey droplet when the red reflex is observed.[1]

The keratometer is an important tool for diagnosing keratoconus. The initial keratometric sign of keratoconus is absence of parallelism of the mires. As the cornea advances, the mires appear smaller. To extend the range of the keratometer, an ancillary lens is placed on the front of the keratometer. If a +1.25 D lens is used, this extends the range to 60 D. To record a reading, 8 D is added to the drum reading (for example, if the drum reads 45 D, adding 8 D yields an actual reading of 53 D). A +2.25 D lens extends the range to 68 D by adding 16 D to the reading.

The photokeratoscope or Placido's disk can provide an overview of the cornea and show the relative steepness of any corneal area. Figure 2-1 depicts a spherical cornea, Figure 2-2 a with-the-rule astigmatic cornea, and Figure 2-3 a keratoconic cornea. The even separation of the rings in the spherical and the astigmatic cornea and the uneven spacing of the rings (especially inferiorly) in the keratoconic cornea should be noted.

Preliminary studies by Maguire and Bourne[30] indicated that using computed corneal topography to identify subtle inferior corneal steepening is highly sensitive for detecting early keratoconus (Plate 5). However, the reliability of such diagnostic topography has not been systematically evaluated clinically, and most practitioners do not have these expensive devices. For example, Mandell and Shie[31] have documented a videokeratographic value of 57.79 D for a keratoconus patient's decentered corneal apex in primary gaze. Upon changing the patient's fixation to center the keratoconic corneal apex, the value was

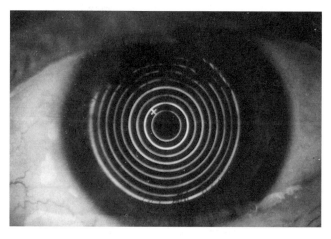

FIGURE 2-1 Spherical cornea.

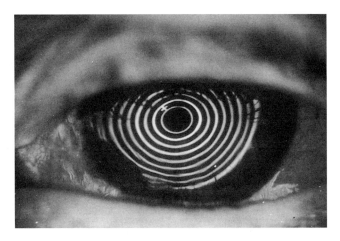

FIGURE 2-2 With-the-rule astigmatic cornea.

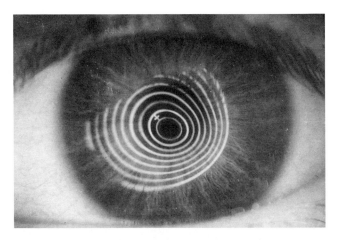

FIGURE 2-3 Keratoconic cornea.

76.70 D. This illustrates the limitations of currently available software for evaluating an irregular corneal surface.

The biomicroscope is a valuable tool. Many classic signs of keratoconus can be observed only with this instrument.

Fleischer's Ring

The Fleischer's ring is a yellow-brown to olive-green ring of pigment that may or may not completely surround the cone's base (Figure 2-4). This ring is formed when hemosiderin (iron) pigment is deposited deep in the epithelium.[6,7] Locating this ring may be made easier by using a cobalt filter and carefully focusing on the epithelium. Once located, the ring should be viewed in white light to assess its extent.

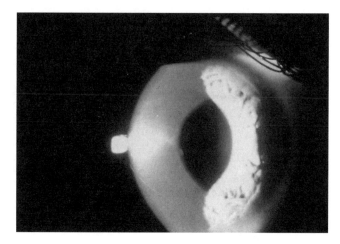

FIGURE 2-4 Fleischer's ring.

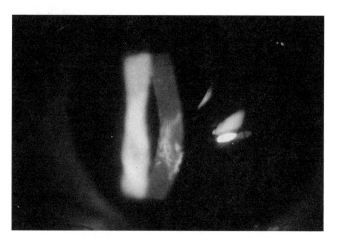

FIGURE 2-5 Lines of Vogt.

Lines of Vogt

Lines of Vogt are small brushlike lines that are generally vertical, but can be oblique. These lines can be found in the keratoconic stroma's deep layers (Figure 2-5) and form along the meridian of greatest curvature;[6] the lines disappear when gentle pressure is exerted on the globe through the lid. Lines of Vogt are more easily viewed when they reappear after pressure is removed. In advanced keratoconus, posterior corneal folds also may be present.

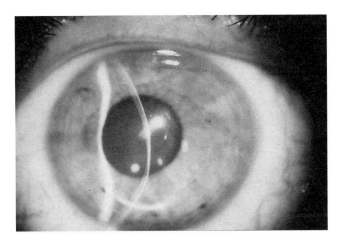

FIGURE 2-6 Corneal thinning.

Corneal Thinning

The normal cornea is about .5 mm thick. Keratoconus patients show clinically significant thinning (e.g., .37 mm) in the disease's advanced stages (Figure 2-6), and a diagnostic criterion based on comparison of central and peripheral corneal thickness has been proposed.[32] Additionally, as the disease progresses, the cone is often displaced inferiorly.[30,33]

Corneal Scarring

Corneal scarring may occur as keratoconus progresses because of ruptures in Bowman's membrane, which then fills with connective tissue.[28] This process is generally not seen in early keratoconus. It also has been reported that flat-fitting contact lenses may accelerate corneal scarring.[34]

Corneal Nerves

Thickening of the corneal nerves makes them more visible in keratoconus.

Swirl Staining

Swirl staining may occur in patients who have never worn contact lenses because basal epithelial cells drop out and the epithelium slides from the periphery as the cornea regenerates.[35-37] Thus a hurricane, vortex, or swirl stain may occur (Figure 2-7). Swirl staining also may result from flat-fitting contact lenses. When this is the case, the lens is generally too flat. A steeper lens often diminishes staining.

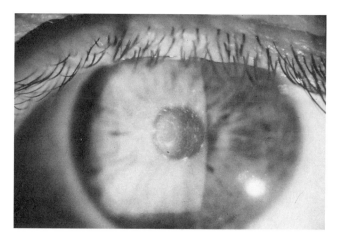

FIGURE 2-7   Swirl staining. (Courtesy Dr. Lisa Badowski.)

CLINICAL PEARL

Swirl staining may occur in patients who have never worn contact lenses because basal epithelial cells drop out and the epithelium slides from the periphery as the cornea regenerates.

Hydrops

Corneal hydrops occurs when the endothelium and Descemet's membrane rupture, aqueous flows into the cornea, and the endothelium reseals. Keratoconus patients who are having an acute episode of corneal hydrops report a sudden loss of vision and a visible white spot on the cornea. Corneal hydrops causes edema and opacification. As the endothelium regenerates, edema and opacification diminish.[28,38] Occasionally hydrops can benefit keratoconus patients who have extremely steep corneas. If the cornea scars, a flatter cornea often results. This flattening may make the cornea easier to fit with a contact lens. Hydrops generally occurs in advanced keratoconus. In addition, an increased incidence of hydrops has been reported in keratoconus patients with Down syndrome.[39]

Munson's Sign

Munson's sign is readily observable without the slit lamp. This sign occurs in advanced keratoconus when the cornea protrudes enough to angulate the lower lid during inferior gaze.[7]

Classification

Keratoconus can be classified by shape,[12,40] central keratometric reading,[12] or progression.[7,8,12] The simplest classification systems are based on keratometric reading or shape (Box 2-1).

Box 2-1
Classification of Keratoconus

Based on severity of curvature

Mild	<45 D in both meridians
Moderate	45 D to 52 D in both meridians
Advanced	>52 D in both meridians
Severe	>62 D in both meridians

Based on shape of cone

Nipple	Small diameter; easiest to fit with contact lenses
Oval	Large diameter; often displaced inferiorly; more difficult to fit
Globus	Largest diameter; 75% of cornea affected; most difficult to fit

---

By using these two classification systems, most cones can be described in terms of severity of curvature and shape (for example, an advanced oval cone).

Contact Lens Design

A number of contact lens designs for patients with keratoconus have been suggested. The advantages and disadvantages of the major lens designs are discussed in the following sections.

Three Point Touch Design

The three point touch design is the classical design used to fit contact lenses for keratoconus. It is the most popular and most frequently advocated design.[41,42] The diameter of the three point touch lens is generally 7.8 mm to 8.5 mm. The three point touch refers to the support provided for the lens by an area of central bearing and two other areas of bearing at the corneal midperiphery, usually in the horizontal meridian.[1] The area of central bearing is about 2 mm to 3 mm in diameter (Figure 2-8).[29,40-42]

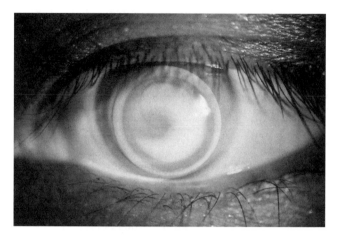

FIGURE 2-8   Acceptable three point touch pattern.

These three areas of bearing distribute the lens' weight across the cornea and prevent lens rocking because of an excessively flat fit. This lens type works well for a cornea with a centrally located cone. Care must be taken to avoid peripheral seal-off and lack of movement. In addition, apical bearing should not exceed 2 mm to 3 mm because increased bearing may cause punctate staining or corneal erosion.[34] In fitting large-diameter cones or cones that are greatly displaced inferiorly, the three point touch design with small lenses cannot be used because poor lens centration usually occurs.

Apical Clearance

This design should result in a lens that vaults the cornea and clears the apex (Figure 2-9). Korb et al[34] proposed that apical bearing may increase the rate of corneal scarring or abrasion and suggested that apical clearance designs cause less trauma to the cornea. Apical clearance lenses are small in diameter (8.0 mm) and have small optic zones (5.8 mm). The apical clearance method works well on cones that have central apexes or on displaced apexes that are only slightly inferior to the visual axis. This method is best applied to smaller cones and is impractical for large cones such as a sagging oval cone or globus cone. A possible disadvantage is reduced visual acuity accompanying apical clearance.[7,43]

Aspheric

Aspheric lenses have been recommended for fitting keratoconus patients. Spherical lenses have a constant radius of curvature in the optic zone and different curvatures cut into the lens in the peripheral areas. However, aspheric lenses gradually flatten from the center to the periphery. The eccentricity or "e value" determines the rate of

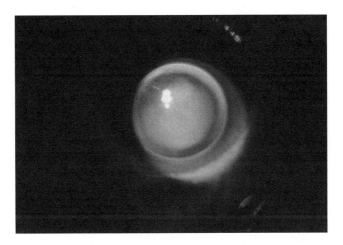

FIGURE 2-9 Apical clearance lens design.

flattening and is independent of the base curve. An average cornea's "e value " is about .65. Decreasing the lens' "e value" decreases the rate of flattening, and increasing the "e value" increases the rate of flattening. When fitting an aspheric lens, good centration is desirable because poorly centered lenses may induce astigmatism and reduce visual acuity. The fluorescein pattern should show central alignment or slight central bearing. The peripheral system should show clearance and lens movement should be apparent. In theory, this approach is ideal; in practice, it may be less than ideal. Problems occur in finding the correct "e value" for the cornea and in reproducing the lens. Examples of this type of lens are the VFL and Ellip-see-con.

Large, Flat Lens

This lens design is useful for displaced apexes.[7,12] As keratoconus develops, the cornea's apex is generally displaced inferiorly. Depending on the cone's steepness, size, or location, a small lens design can be impractical. If a small lens is placed on an inferiorly displaced apex, the lens is generally positioned low, and the lid often dislocates the lens with each blink. In such cases a lens of larger diameter (9.0 mm to 10.0 mm) is preferable. The fitting method positions the lens' upper edge under the upper lid to prevent lens dislocation (Figure 2-10). The peripheral system must be flat enough—typically 1 mm to 2 mm flatter than standard lens designs— to permit lens movement. Often a large lens is too steep peripherally and binds the peripheral cornea. In contrast, a very flat lens without secondary bearing often rocks and is uncomfortable. Large flat lenses result in a larger area of bearing than lenses fitted using the three point touch design and thus may be more prone to erosion or scarring.[1,7,11,34]

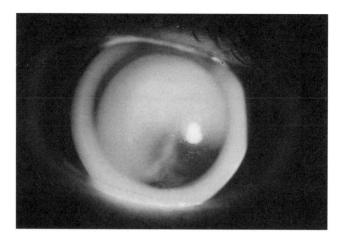

FIGURE 2-10 Large flat lid attachment fit.

Keratoconus Lens Systems

Many lens systems exist for fitting keratoconus patients. Often these systems use a cookbook approach and suggest that lens diameter be increased as the cone develops. However, we prefer lenses with apical clearance or minimal apical bearing in advanced keratoconus unless the apex is decentered or large.

Soper Lens System

The objective of the Soper lens system, popularized by Soper and Jarrett,[44] is based on sagittal depth. The principle behind this system is that a constant base curve with an increased diameter results in increased sagittal depth and a steeper lens. The lenses included in the fitting set are categorized as mild (7.5 mm diameter, 6.0 mm optic zone diameter), moderate (8.5 mm diameter, 7.0 mm optic zone diameter), and advanced (9.5 mm diameter, 8.0 mm optic zone diameter). The initial trial lens is selected based on the cone's degree of advancement (Figure 2-11).[45] The more advanced the cone, the larger the diameter of the recommended lens; the smaller and more centrally located the apex, the smaller the lens' diameter. Soper[46] stated that when properly manufactured, his lens is not a bicurve lens but incorporates the following curvatures: a 26 D curve (0.2 mm wide) initially generated using a diamond tool; a 37 D curve (0.2 mm wide) generated using a velveteen tool; and a 40 D curve (0.1 mm wide) generated using a velveteen tool. When carefully manufactured, these curves all blend together. However, many laboratories inappropriately manufacture this lens as a bicurve lens with a peripheral system that may be too steep. The secondary curve (7.5 mm and 45 D) remains the same regardless of whether the base curve is 52 D or 62 D. When central

Soper Keratoconus Diagnostic Set

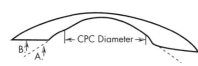

This record curve used on each lens A. (43.00 or 45.00) is to facilitate the placement in that area of the paraboic peripheral and intermediate curves which creates a "ski-like" configuration B. to fit over the flat peripheal area of the cornea. The diameter of the CPC is critical as it is used to calculate the sagittal depth of the lens.

		Sagittal depth (mm)	CPC (D)	Power (D)	Lens diameter mm	Thickness (mm)	CPC diameter (oz mm)
Moderate cone	Try first						
	A	0.68	48.00/43.00	-4.5	7.5	0.10	6.0
	B	0.73	52.00/45.00	-8.50	7.5	0.10	6.0
	C	0.80	56.00/45.00	-12.50	7.5	0.10	6.0
	D	0.87	60.00/45.00	-16.50	7.5	0.10	6.0
Advanced cone	Try first						
	E	1.00	52.00/45.00	-8.50	8.5	0.10	7.0
	F	1.12	56.00/45.00	-12.50	8.5	0.10	7.0
	G	1.22	60.00/45.00	-16.50	8.5	0.10	7.0
Severe cone	Try first						
	H	1.37	52.00/45.00	-8.50	9.5	0.10	8.0
	I	1.52	56.00/45.00	-12.50	9.5	0.10	8.0
	J	1.67	60.00/45.00	-16.50	9.5	0.10	8.0

FIGURE 2-11 Soper lens system.

alignment is achieved, the periphery is often too tight, resulting in inadequate lens movement and tear exchange and the need to modify (flatten) the lens periphery.

McGuire Lens System

The McGuire keratoconic system is a modification of the Soper lens design (Table 2-1). In the McGuire system, fitting sets are categorized as nipple (8.1 mm diameter, 5.5 mm optic zone), oval (8.6 mm diameter, 6 mm optic zone), or globus (9.1 mm diameter, 6.5 mm optic zone).[47] The McGuire system has four peripheral curves; the three inner curves are each .3 mm wide and the peripheral curve is .4 mm wide. From most central to most peripheral, the curves are 3 D (.5 mm), 9 D (1.5 mm), 17 D (3 mm), and 27 D (5 mm) flatter than the base curve. This lens system allows adequate edge clearance and movement.

NiCone Lens

The NiCone lens system (available from Lancaster Contact Lens Co., Lancaster, Pennsylvania) is promoted as having three base curves and one constant peripheral curve of 12.25 mm. NiCone fitting sets are designated by the numbers one to three. The Number 1 cone set is for

TABLE 2-1

McGuire Lens Fitting Sets

Base Curve	Power	Diameter	Optic Zone	Peripheral Curves 1st	2nd	3rd	4th
Oval-Cone Fitting Set:							
50.00	−8.00	8.6	6.0	47.00/.3	41.00/.3	33.00/.3	23.00/.4
51.00	−8.00	8.6	6.0	48.00/.3	42.00/.3	34.00/.3	24.00/.4
52.00	−10.00	8.6	6.0	49.00/.3	43.00/.3	35.00/.3	25.00/.4
53.00	−10.00	8.6	6.0	50.00/.3	44.00/.3	36.00/.3	26.00/.4
54.00	−12.00	8.6	6.0	51.00/.3	45.00/.3	37.00/.3	27.00/.4
55.00	−12.00	8.6	6.0	52.00/.3	46.00/.3	38.00/.3	28.00/.4
56.00	−14.00	8.6	6.0	53.00/.3	47.00/.3	39.00/.3	29.00/.4
57.00	−14.00	8.6	6.0	54.00/.3	48.00/.3	40.00/.3	30.00/.4
58.00	−16.00	8.6	6.0	55.00/.3	49.00/.3	41.00/.3	31.00/.4
59.00	−16.00	8.6	6.0	56.00/.3	50.00/.3	42.00/.3	32.00/.4
60.00	−18.00	8.6	6.0	57.00/.3	51.00/.3	43.00/.3	33.00/.4
61.00	−18.00	8.6	6.0	58.00/.3	52.00/.3	44.00/.3	34.00/.4
Nipple-Cone Fitting Set:							
50.00	−8.00	8.1	5.5	47.00/.3	41.00/.3	33.00/.3	23.00/.4
52.00	−10.00	8.1	5.5	49.00/.3	43.00/.3	35.00/.3	25.00/.4
54.00	−12.00	8.1	5.5	51.00/.3	45.00/.3	37.00/.3	27.00/.4
56.00	−14.00	8.1	5.5	53.00/.3	47.00/.3	39.00/.3	29.00/.4
58.00	−16.00	8.1	5.5	55.00/.3	49.00/.3	41.00/.3	31.00/.4
60.00	−18.00	8.1	5.5	57.00/.3	51.00/.3	43.00/.3	33.00/.4
Globus-Cone Fitting Set:							
50.00	−8.00	9.1	6.5	47.00/.3	41.00/.3	33.00/.3	23.00/.4
52.00	−10.00	9.1	6.5	49.00/.3	43.00/.3	35.00/.3	25.00.4
54.00	−12.00	9.1	6.5	51.00/.3	45.00/.3	37.00/.3	27.00/.4
56.00	−14.00	9.1	6.5	53.00/.3	47.00/.3	39.00/.3	29.00/.4
58.00	−16.00	9.1	6.5	55.00/.3	49.00/.3	41.00/.3	31.00/.4
60.00	−18.00	9.1	6.5	57.00/.3	51.00/.3	43.00/.3	33.00/.4

Reproduced from Caroline PJ, Doughman DJ, McGuire JR: A new contact lens design for keratoconus: a continuing report, *Cont Lens J* 12:17-20, 1978.

patients with keratometry readings between 40 D and 52 D, the Number 2 set is for patients with keratometry readings from 53 D to 65 D, and the Number 3 set is for patients with keratometry readings greater than 65 D. The preferred lens alignment is feather touch.[48] The second base curve is a 0.3 mm transition zone between the central base curve and the third base curve that rests on the normal peripheral cornea. The manufacturer indicates that "lathe cut, optically polished peripheral base curves prevent optical distortion that ground curvatures create in a lens." In reality, these additional base curves are peripheral curves added to improve lens performance. The lens diameter and other parameters vary depending on lens steepness. A disadvantage of this system is that the values the manufacturer uses for the peripheral curvatures are unknown because of patented design; not knowing the lens' curvatures in the peripheral areas limits the practitioner's ability to modify the lens and makes the practitioner dependent on the laboratory for fitting design changes.

Soft Lens and Combination Lens Alternatives

Soft lenses and combination lens alternatives have been advocated for keratoconus patients.

Hydrogel Lenses

Soft contact lenses are used to fit keratoconus patients who cannot tolerate rigid lenses or who have early disease.[49,50] The main advantage of these lenses is greater comfort. A soft lens may partially correct irregular astigmatism and thus permit spectacle overcorrection. Power to reduce anisometropia also can be placed in the soft lens. The disadvantages of soft lenses include reduced visual acuity and the need for spectacle overcorrection for best visual acuity.

Specialized soft lenses also can be used in keratoconus. Because these lenses are extremely thick (.3 mm to .5 mm), they sometimes correct the irregular astigmatism of keratoconus as effectively as rigid lenses. This lens design is most often indicated for patients for whom a rigid lens cannot be fitted because of severe apical displacement, an extremely steep cone, or a cone of particularly large diameter. In such cases the hydrogel lens' large diameter (14 mm to 15 mm) allows it to bear on the sclera and the corneal apex (Figure 2-12), enabling the lens to center, which may not be possible with smaller rigid lenses. One custom-made soft lens for keratoconus, manufactured by Flexlens, Inc. (Englewood, Colorado), is made of a 45% water content

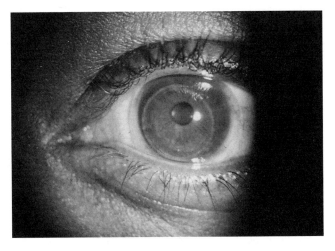

FIGURE 2-12   Flexlens soft cone lens.

material and can be made in any power or curvature. When high molecular weight fluorescein is instilled in the eye of a patient wearing this lens, the fluorescein pattern under the lens is similar to that of a rigid lens. Lens movement is vital for successful fit. Lens movement can be maximized by varying the secondary curve.

Another soft cone lens is the Fre-Flex Cone Lens (Optech, Inc., Englewood, Colorado). This lens design is based on sagittal depth. The lens' base curve (8.4 mm) and diameter (14 mm) are held constant and the optic zone diameter (OZD) is varied to produce different fitting relations. The larger the OZD, the more steeply fitting the lens. These lenses, which are made of a 55% water content material, are manufactured in three sizes: Cone A (5.9 mm OZD), Cone B (6.9 mm OZD), and Cone C (7.9 mm OZD). The Cone A lens, although the flattest, is often successful in correcting even steep cones and should be tried before the steeper Cone B and C lenses. Disadvantages of the Flexlens and Fre-Flex Cone lenses include corneal edema and neovascularization.

Piggyback Lens Designs

A piggyback lens system consists of a rigid lens fitted on top of a soft lens.[51] Indications for this technique include rigid lens intolerance and mechanical problems such as recurrent corneal erosion. The combination of rigid and soft lenses results in visual acuity equal to that achieved by using a rigid lens alone.[52] Because the soft lens decreases the corneal curvature difference between the central and the peripheral cornea, the base curve of the rigid lens used with the soft lens is often flatter than the base curve of a rigid lens alone. Only materials with high oxygen transmissibility should be used for both components.

CLINICAL PEARL

Indications for the piggyback system include rigid lens intolerance and mechanical problems such as recurrent corneal erosion.

The soft lens must move adequately in piggyback systems. If the soft lens binds, the patient may have problems. The rigid gas-permeable lens should have minimal center and edge thickness to promote centration and comfort, and a rounded edge to prevent tearing of the soft lens. To evaluate the rigid lens' fit, the presence and location of any oxygen bubbles under the rigid lens should be noted. Central bubbles indicate a steep lens; bubbles near the lens edge indicate a flat fit. Patients should use soft contact lens solutions with a piggyback system. Many rigid lens solutions contain preservatives that may be toxic to the cornea in high concentrations, and soft lenses may absorb these solutions.

Piggyback systems are usually used in difficult cases but are not the preferred lens system for keratoconus. Long-term care for two types of lenses is often difficult. Wearing time should be carefully monitored in these instances.

Another type of piggyback system is the countersunk lens, available from Flexlens, Inc., (Figures 2-13 and 2-14).[53] This countersunk lens is a thick soft lens, 14.5 mm to 15 mm in diameter, with a groove cut into it. A rigid lens is fitted into this groove. The rigid lens is designed so that the lens' thickness plus the tear reservoir is equal to the groove depth. If the rigid lens is too thick, it protrudes from the groove and may be blinked out; if the rigid lens is too thin, the whole system may dislocate if the lid catches the groove during blinking. To permit tear exchange, the rigid lens should be made .1 mm to .2 mm smaller than the groove diameter. The rigid lens fit is evaluated by observing the location of any oxygen bubbles. The system's main objective is to center a rigid lens on a displaced corneal apex. Major disadvantages of countersunk piggyback lenses are the inconvenience of a two lens system, corneal edema, neovascularization, and tearing of the soft lens at the groove junction.

Flexlens piggyback lens

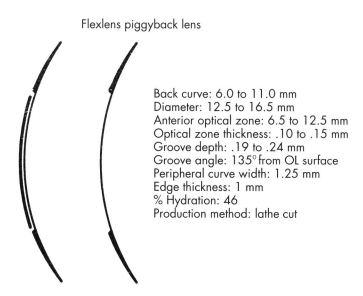

Back curve: 6.0 to 11.0 mm
Diameter: 12.5 to 16.5 mm
Anterior optical zone: 6.5 to 12.5 mm
Optical zone thickness: .10 to .15 mm
Groove depth: .19 to .24 mm
Groove angle: 135° from OL surface
Peripheral curve width: 1.25 mm
Edge thickness: 1 mm
% Hydration: 46
Production method: lathe cut

FIGURE 2-13 Countersunk piggyback lens system. (From Caroline PJ, Doughman DJ: A new piggyback lens design for the correction of irregular astigmatism: a preliminary report, *Cont Lens J* 13:39-42 [53], 1979.)

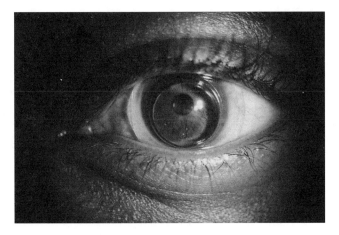

FIGURE 2-14   Countersunk piggyback lens system.

SoftPerm Lens

The SoftPerm lens (from Pilkington/Barnes-Hind, Sunnyvale, California) is a hybrid lens with a rigid gas-permeable center surrounded by a soft hydrophilic skirt. This lens may be indicated for patients with displaced corneal apexes or for patients who cannot tolerate rigid lenses. Advantages of the lens include its one piece design, better centration on displaced apexes, and improved comfort compared to rigid gas-permeable lenses. However, the SoftPerm lens has limitations. Most early keratoconus patients can be successfully fitted with rigid lenses. For patients with advanced keratoconus, in which a lens of larger diameter is useful, the lens often fits tight, which results in limited movement. In addition, the lens material has a low Dk value (rigid portion, 14 Dk; soft portion, 5.5 Dk). The major problems associated with this lens are difficult handling, lack of lens movement, corneal edema, and neovascularization.

Fitting Procedure

Information on the diagnosis of and fitting methods for keratoconus has been presented. A specific procedure to facilitate fitting or refitting the keratoconus patient follows.

Keratometry

Although keratometric readings may be of limited use in fitting keratoconus patients, they can assist in initial trial lens selection and in documenting disease progression. The keratometric range should be extended as necessary.

Refraction

Careful refraction is mandatory. Patients with keratoconus often have unpredictably good best-corrected visual acuity. Large amounts of cylinder, frequently at an increasingly oblique axis, are sometimes found. Retinoscopic and keratometric results are excellent starting points for determining subjective refraction. Careful refinement of cylinder axis and avoidance of overminusing are necessary. Accurate refraction provides a baseline best visual acuity without contact lenses, serving as a reference point for expected acuity after correction by contact lenses. The corrected acuity should be at least as good as that achieved with spectacles. Prescriptions are often based on subjective refraction results to provide backup spectacles for patients who wear contact lenses, or as the primary correction for patients who cannot wear contact lenses.

Trial Lens Fitting

Trial lens fitting is important for patients with keratoconus (Table 2-2). No formula exists for predicting proper lens fit. The initial trial lens should have a base curve that either splits the two keratometric readings or is slightly flatter than the mean corneal curvature. If the patient has never worn contact lenses, instilling a topical corneal

TABLE 2-2
Burger Keratoconus Trial Lens Set Using Oxyflow F3O

| Secondary curve | | | Primary curve | | | Base curve | | |
Base curve	Base curve radius	Power	Diameter	Optic Zone Diameter	Width	Blend*	Width	Thickness
61.00	5.53	−16.00	8.0	5.8	7.5/.6	8.5	9.5/.4	.15
60.00	5.63	−15.00	8.0	5.8	7.5/.6	8.5	9.5/.4	.15
59.00	5.72	−14.00	8.0	5.8	7.5/.6	8.5	9.5/.4	.15
58.00	5.82	−14.00	8.0	5.8	8.0/.6	9.0	10.0/.4	.15
57.00	5.92	−12.00	8.0	5.8	8.0/.6	9.0	10.0/.4	.15
56.00	6.03	−12.00	8.0	5.8	8.0/.6	9.0	10.0/.4	.15
55.00	6.14	−12.00	8.4	6.2	8.0/.6	9.0	10.0/.4	.15
54.00	6.24	−11.00	8.4	6.2	8.0/.6	9.0	10.0/.4	.15
53.00	6.37	−10.00	8.4	6.2	8.5/.6	9.5	10.5/.4	.15
52.00	6.49	−10.00	8.4	6.2	8.5/.6	9.5	10.5/.4	.15
51.00	6.62	−8.00	8.4	6.2	8.5/.6	9.5	10.5/.4	.15
50.00	6.75	−7.00	8.4	6.2	8.5/.6	9.5	10.5/.4	.15
49.00	6.89	−6.00	8.4	6.2	8.5/.6	9.5	10.5/.4	.15
48.00	7.03	−5.00	8.4	6.2	8.5/.6	9.5	10.5/.4	.15
47.00	7.18	−4.00	8.4	6.2	8.5/.6	9.5	10.5/.4	.15

*Allow .1 mm for medium blend.

anesthetic will reduce reflex tearing and help the practitioner obtain more accurate refractive endpoint and visual acuity measurements.

CLINICAL PEARL

The initial trial lens should have a base curve that either splits the two keratometric readings or is slightly flatter than the mean corneal curvature.

Fluorescein Pattern Analysis

The ideal keratoconic fluorescein pattern depends on the lens design chosen. The authors prefer to use a minimum apical clearance design whenever possible. The pattern should show slight fluorescein pooling in the center and a narrow band of touch in the intermediate curve area. In addition, the peripheral curve should be flat enough to allow a reservoir of tears to collect. This combination aids tear interchange and movement. The three point touch design produces a similar pattern except for the central 2 mm to 3 mm of bearing.

To analyze the fit, the fluorescein pattern should be divided into two areas: the central portion (including the entire area under the optic zone) and the peripheral zone. Each area should be analyzed separately. The location and amount of bearing should be observed. If central bearing is found, the lens should be steepened if an apical clearance pattern is desired. If pooling in the periphery is absent, the peripheral system should be flatter (Figure 2-15). If insufficient lens movement and excessive bearing in the area of the secondary curves are found, then the secondary curve is too steep and is preventing

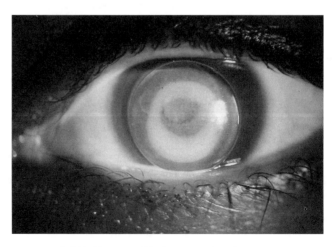

FIGURE 2-15 Tight peripheral curve.

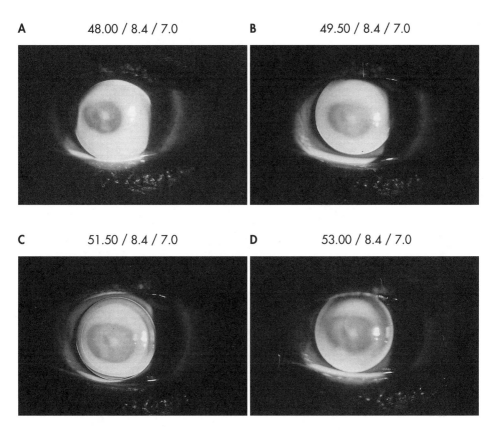

A 48.00 / 8.4 / 7.0

B 49.50 / 8.4 / 7.0

C 51.50 / 8.4 / 7.0

D 53.00 / 8.4 / 7.0

FIGURE 2-16 **A** to **H,** Series of contact lenses showing base curve (BC), diameter (Dia), and optic zone diameter (OZD).

lens movement. Absence of fluorescein in the secondary or peripheral area can result when the lens seals off. Location, size, and persistence of air bubbles under the lens should be carefully noted. A central air bubble may indicate that the lens is too steep. In contrast, paracentral air bubbles may indicate that the optic zone is too large. Figure 2-16 shows a series of trial lenses in which the base curve increases while the diameter and optic zone are kept relatively constant. Note the decrease in central bearing and peripheral edge lift, and the increase in intermediate touch as the base curve increases.

Corneal apex position relative to the trial lens should be determined. In general, the lower the apex, the larger the lens diameter required for centration. A low-riding lens may be too flat or too small. A larger lens may be required for centration. In attempting to fit a larger lens, a lid attachment fit is desirable (Figure 2-10); however, the peripheral system must be flat enough to prevent paracentral seal-off that could result in decreased movement and tear exchange. If adequate centration cannot be achieved, a soft cone lens should be

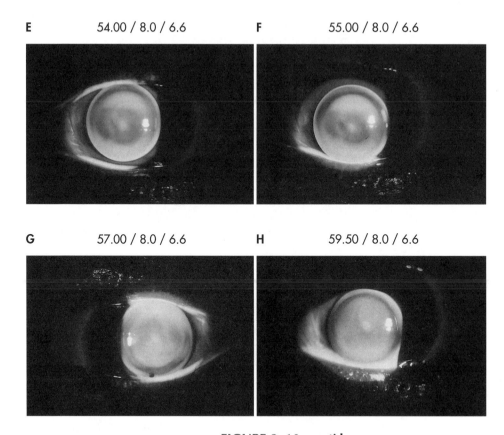

| E | 54.00 / 8.0 / 6.6 | F | 55.00 / 8.0 / 6.6 |
| G | 57.00 / 8.0 / 6.6 | H | 59.50 / 8.0 / 6.6 |

FIGURE 2-16, cont'd

considered. Fitting such specialty lenses requires a trial set, and this lens should be regarded as a last resort.

Each trial lens should be allowed to settle on the eye for about 10 to 20 minutes before evaluation. Keratoconic corneas are very pliable, and if the patient previously wore flat lenses, the degree of corneal molding can be marked. Figures 2-17 through 2-19 depict the corneal change that occurs when a steeper lens is placed on the eye and allowed adequate time to settle.

Trial lens overrefractions should be compared: each system's total power should be about equal. This comparison is important for evaluating the consistency of the diagnostic lenses (Box 2-2).

Box 2-2 Comparison of Trial Lens Overrefractions

Base Curve	Power	Overrefraction	Net Power
50.00	−10.00	−3.00	−13.00
52.00	−11.00	−4.00	−15.00

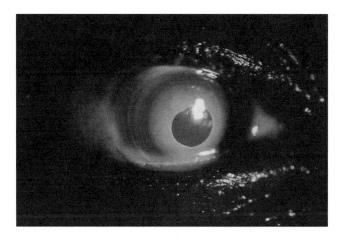

FIGURE 2-17 Initial view of 6.25 base curve after removal of 7.35 base curve.

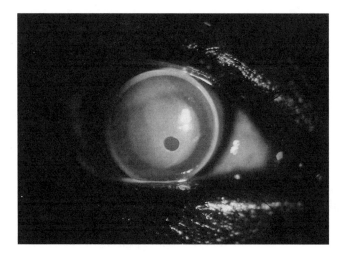

FIGURE 2-18 View after 20 minutes.

Steepening the base curve by 2.00 D creates a fluid lens of +2.00 D. To compensate for this effect, an equal amount of minus power (that is, −2.00 D) must be added. Therefore a lens with the parameters 50.00/−13.00 is theoretically equivalent to a 52.00/−15.00 lens.

Once adequate fit is achieved, a manufacturing laboratory must be chosen to make the lens according to specifications. Some laboratories have a standard keratoconic lens design, but these lenses are often too steep peripherally. If the ordered lens looks different from the diagnostic trial lens, modification in the office or laboratory is necessary. Manufacturing a trial lens set according to specifications is important to ensure a standard for comparison during fitting and in checking

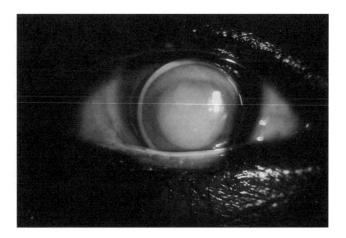

FIGURE 2-19 View after 40 minutes.

ordered lenses. A gas-permeable material with medium oxygen trans-missibility (range 12 to 39 DK) is optimal. This choice allows ample oxygen and is less prone to warping and dryness.

Problem Solving

The practitioner must often solve contact lens fitting problems for keratoconus patients. These problems include lack of lens movement, reduced visual acuity, poor lens centration, and corneal staining. Successful fitting depends upon solving these problems.

Lack of Contact Lens Movement

Lack of lens movement (also termed lens binding) may be caused by peripheral curve seal-off, secondary curve seal-off, or a sharp junction at the optic zone border.

CLINICAL PEARL

Lack of lens movement may be caused by peripheral curve seal-off, secondary curve seal-off, or a sharp junction at the optic zone border.

Peripheral curve seal-off occurs when the peripheral curve is too steep, causing the lens to bind at the edge and preventing lens movement and tear interchange (see Figure 2-15). Keratoconus is a disease of the central cornea and usually does not affect the peripheral

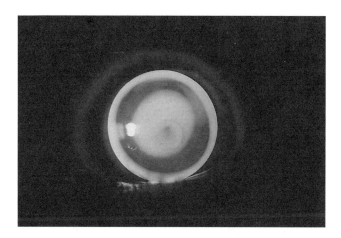

FIGURE 2-20 Wide and tight intermediate curve.

cornea's curvature; the peripheral curvature radii of the contact lens should be chosen accordingly. For example, a normal cornea (43.00 D to 43.50 D) requires peripheral lens curvature of about 10.5 mm. However, many manufacturers use much steeper peripheral curves for keratoconic lenses; the resulting lens does not have adequate edge lift and binds to the cornea. This problem can be corrected by specifying flatter peripheral curves when ordering the lens.

The second most common reason for lack of lens movement is a too-steep secondary curve. Adequate edge lift is evident in the fluorescein pattern from pooling (which indicates a tear reservoir) and a large intermediate (or secondary) bearing area (Figure 2-20). In such cases lens movement is restricted by the tight intermediate area. The secondary curve is too steep or too wide, preventing fluid interchange and lens movement. This deficiency is corrected by using flatter curvature or increasing the peripheral curve width.

The third reason for lack of lens movement is a sharp junction between the secondary curve and base curve at the optic zone border. The lens seals and may cause discomfort and epithelial erosion. This problem is remedied by blending this area heavily so that the lens has a rounded junction to increase lens movement.

Reduced Visual Acuity

Another problem in keratoconus patients is reduced visual acuity even with contact lens correction. This reduced acuity may result from incorrect power, corneal scarring, or astigmatism that is either residual or from lens flexure.

A common reason for reduced visual acuity (besides scarring) is overminusing. In fitting keratoconus patients, many practitioners prescribe too much minus correction. Overminusing may occur because a patient has not adapted to the lenses and is tearing profusely, and thus accepts more minus correction than is necessary. Overrefraction at follow-up visits is essential to check the system's power as patients adapt.

A second cause of reduced visual acuity is corneal scarring that occurs in the visual axis.[54] The denser the scarring, the greater the reduction in visual acuity. Corneal scarring may be minimized by fitting lenses with apical clearance.[34]

Astigmatism also may reduce visual acuity. This effect may take one of two forms: lens flexure or residual astigmatism. Keratoconus lenses are steep and high-powered; if too thin, the lenses may flex. Lens flexure, manifesting as residual astigmatism,[55] can be measured by performing overkeratometry. If flexure is absent, the keratometric reading is spherical; if flexure is present, the keratometric reading is not spherical. Using a thicker lens and a moderately oxygen-transmissible lens instead of a highly oxygen-transmissible lens helps prevent lens flexure. The higher the oxygen transmissibility, the softer the material and the more the lens flexes.

Residual astigmatism, like lens flexure, occurs while the lens is in place. However, overkeratometry readings are spherical in residual astigmatism, but not in lens flexure. In this case residual astigmatism is caused by the crystalline lens or, more often, the corneal surface. The easiest and best way to correct residual astigmatism is to prescribe spectacles with the necessary power.

Poor Lens Centration

Another problem in fitting keratoconus patients is poor lens centration, caused by a decentered corneal apex or an extremely flat-fitting lens. The steeper the cornea becomes, the more decentered (usually inferiorly) the apex becomes, and the more difficult it is to fit a contact lens. In these cases the lens often rides low. Moreover, if a small lens is fitted to a decentered apex, the lens may become decentered when the patient blinks. In such cases a larger, flatter lens can be used to create a lid attachment fit.[56]

Excessively flat-fitting lenses also may cause poor lens centration. A lens may be so flat that it rocks on the corneal apex and never establishes a proper fit. When the patient blinks, the lens may decenter and pop out. In such cases the contact lens fit must be steepened appropriately by conducting a complete diagnostic trial lens fitting. Ample settling time after each trial lens insertion must be allowed before viewing the resultant fluorescein fitting pattern. Diagnostic fitting may take 1 to 2 hours to neutralize the effects of previous contact lenses. New lenses may be substantially steeper if diagnostic lenses are given ample time to settle.

Corneal Staining

Another cause for concern is corneal staining (either central or peripheral). Peripheral staining may occur because of tight peripheral curves, poor blending, dryness, or partial blinking.

Tight peripheral curves result in staining at the lens' edges and a lens indentation mark. These problems can be corrected by using flatter, better blended peripheral and secondary curves. Staining of the peripheral cornea (at 3 to 9 o'clock) also may be present because of dryness or partial blinking. Edge improvements, lubricants, and blinking exercises should be prescribed as necessary.

Modification

In fitting keratoconus patients, lens modification is crucial. Returning the contact lens to the manufacturer for modification is often impossible. A patient who requires a lens with parameters of 50.00/−16.00 cannot see without the lens. Plates 6 through 8 depict a contact lens with a tight peripheral system, its imprint on the cornea, and the lens fit after modification.

Many different modification units are available, but one with multiple spindles for polishing and cutting is the most efficient. A more extensive selection of tools, especially for steep curvature, is necessary for modifying keratoconus lenses. For major modification, diamond-impregnated brass tools are recommended. The range in tool size provided should be 7.5 mm to 11.0 mm (45.00 D to 30.75 D), progressing in 0.5 mm steps. To polish the rough cut, polishing laps with radii of 6.60 mm to 12.00 mm (51.00 D to 27.00 D) are suggested. The difference in laps should be .15 mm at the steep end (6.60 mm to 7.50 mm), .5 mm to 1 mm at the flat end (9.0 mm to 12.0 mm), and 0.2 mm to 0.5 mm in the normal corneal curvature range (7.8 mm to 9.0 mm). These size ranges for diamond tools and polishing laps should accomplish most secondary and peripheral curve modifications. A polishing lap that is steeper than the diamond tool is often necessary to completely remove the tool marks.

Referral Criteria

In 15% to 20% of the keratoconic population, a corneal transplant is eventually required.[2,3] The patient should be referred for transplant if any of the following generally accepted referral criteria are met:

1. Contact lens intolerance. The patient cannot wear the lens, even if the lens fit looks adequate.

2. Inability to fit the patient with a contact lens. The patient can tolerate a contact lens, but an acceptable lens cannot be fitted.

3. Decreased vision (generally from scarring) that prevents the patient from doing necessary visual tasks. The patient wants to wear lenses, and does so successfully, but the decreased vision (generally secondary to scarring) causes him or her problems in performing necessary visual tasks. For some patients this may occur at an acuity level of 20/60; for others it may occur at 20/100.

4. A large cone with progressive thinning in the periphery.

5. The danger of perforation. The cornea becomes so thin that a danger exists that it will perforate. This is extremely rare in keratoconus.

All patients should be informed of the long healing process required after corneal transplant. The normal time required for visual rehabilitation is about 9 to 10 months, although visual correction can be prescribed as early as 3 months postoperatively.

Surgical Alternatives

Various types of surgery are available for the patient with keratoconus. Penetrating keratoplasty is the most common.[57] In this procedure the keratoconic cornea is prepared by removing the cornea's central area, and a full thickness corneal button is sutured in its place. Depending on the criteria used to assess the success rate, this surgery is 90% to 95% successful.[3, 58-61] Contact lenses often are required after this procedure for best visual correction. An alternative procedure, lamellar keratoplasty, is not a full thickness corneal transplant, but a partial corneal transplant. The cornea is removed to the depth of Descemet's membrane and the donor button is sutured in place. This technique is technically difficult, and visual acuity is inferior to that obtained after penetrating keratoplasty.[61] As a result, lamellar keratoplasty is largely confined to the treatment of large cones or keratoglobus.[61] This technique requires less recovery time and poses less of a risk for corneal graft rejection.[62] Its disadvantages include vascularization and graft haziness.

In thermokeratoplasty, a hot ring is placed along the cone's base, and the cornea is heated and traumatized. As a result, a corneal scar develops, reduces the corneal curvature, and allows a flatter contact lens to be fitted.[63] This procedure is rarely performed in the United States.[64]

Epikeratoplasty is primarily suited for contact-lens-intolerant patients in whom scarring has not yet occurred.[57, 65] In addition, prospective epikeratoplasty patients must have visual acuity of at

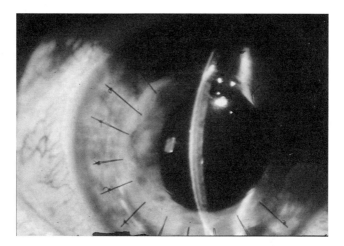

FIGURE 2-21 Epikeratoplasty.

least 20/40 when wearing contact lenses.[57, 65, 66] In this procedure, the central host epithelium is debrided and the donor cornea is sewn over the keratoconic cornea. The donor button is regular in shape and provides the uniform surface necessary for good visual correction (Figure 2-21). Advantages of this procedure include its nonpenetrating nature, retention of the globe's mechanical integrity, and retention of normal host endothelium to avoid graft rejection.[56, 62] Occasionally, contact lenses may be required postoperatively for best visual correction.[64]

Conclusion

Keratoconus presents a great challenge to the optometrist. This disease is best managed by appropriately fitted contact lenses. Information has been provided to allow the practitioner to diagnose keratoconus, to counsel the patient about this condition, to choose the right fitting system, and to decide when surgical consultation is necessary.

References

1. Bennett ES: Keratoconus. In: Bennett ES, Grohe RM, ed: *Rigid gas- permeable contact lenses*, New York, 1986, Professional Press Books, 297-344.
2. Crews MJ, Driebe WT, Stern GA: The clinical management of keratoconus: a 6 year retrospective study, *CLAO* 20:194-197, 1994.
3. Smiddy WE, Hamburg TR, Kracher GP, Stark WJ: Keratoconus: contact lens or keratoplasty?, *Ophthalmol* 95:487-492, 1988.
4. Tuft SJ, Moodaley LC, Gregory WM, Davison CR, Buckley RJ: Prognostic factors for the progression of keratoconus, *Ophthalmol* 101:439-447, 1994.

5. Hofstetter HW: A keratoscopic survey of 13,395 eyes, *Am J Optom Arch Am Acad Optom* 36:3-11, 1959.

6. Duke-Elder S, Leigh AG: Ectatic conditions. Keratoconus (conical cornea). In: Duke-Elder S, Leigh AG, ed: *System of Ophthalmology Vol 8, Part 2: Diseases of the Outer Eye,* St Louis, 1965, Mosby, 964-975.

7. Krachmer JH, Feder RS, Belin MW: Keratoconus and related noninflammatory corneal thinning disorders, *Surv Ophthalmol* 28:293-322, 1984.

8. Reinke AR: Keratoconus: a review of research and current fitting techniques. Part 1, *Int. Cont Lens Clin* 2:66-79, 1975.

9. Kennedy RH, Bourne WM, Dyer JA: A 48-year clinical and epidemiologic study of keratoconus, *Am J Ophthalmol* 101:267-273, 1986.

10. Ridley F: Contact lenses in treatment of keratoconus, *Br J Ophthalmol* 40:295-304, 1956.

11. Hall KGC: A comprehensive study of keratoconus, *Br J Physiol Opt* 20:215-256, 1963.

12. Buxton JN, Keates RH, Hoefle FB: The contact lens correction of keratoconus. In: Dabezies OH, ed: *Contact Lenses: The CLAO Guide to Basic Science and Clinical Practice,* Orlando, 1984, Grune & Stratton, 55.1-55.14.

13. Teng CC: Electron microscope study of the pathology of keratoconus: Part I, *Am J Ophthalmol* 55:18-47, 1963.

14. Newsome DA, Foidart J-M, Hassell JR, Krachmer JH, Rodrigues MM, Katz SI: Detection of certain collagen types in normal and keratoconus corneas, *Inv Ophthalmol Vis Sci* 20:738-750, 1981.

15. Rehany U, Lahav M, Shoshan S: Collagenolytic activity in keratoconus, *Ann Ophthalmol* 14:751-754, 1982.

16. Critchfield JW, Calandra AJ, Nesburn AB, Kenney MC: Keratoconus: I . Biochemical studies, *Exp Eye Res* 46:953-963, 1988.

17. Rabinowitz YS, Garbus J, McDonnell PJ: Computer-assisted corneal topography in family members of patients with keratoconus, *Arch Ophthalmol* 108:365-371, 1990.

18. Hammerstein W: Zur Genetik des Keratoconus [Genetics of conical cornea], *Albrecht Von Graefes Arch Klin Exp Ophthalmol* 190:293-308, 1974.

19. Rahi A, Davies P, Ruben M, Lobascher D, Menon J: Keratoconus and coexisting atopic disease, *Br J Ophthalmol* 61:761-764, 1977.

20. Kemp EG, Lewis CJ: Immunoglobulin pattern in keratoconus with particular reference to total and specific IgE levels, *Br J Ophthalmol* 66:717-720, 1982.

21. Karseras AG, Ruben M: Aetiology of keratoconus, *Br J Ophthalmol* 60:522-525, 1976.

22. Gritz DC, McDonnell PJ: Keratoconus and ocular massage, *Am J Ophthalmol* 106:757-758, 1988.

23. Ing MR: The development of corneal astigmatism in contact lens wearers, *Ann Ophthalmol* 8:309-314, 1976.

24. Hartstein J: Keratoconus that developed in patients wearing corneal contact lenses: report of four cases, *Arch Ophthalmol* 80:345-346, 1968.

25. Steahly LP: Keratoconus following contact lens wear, *Ann Ophthalmol* 10:1177-1179, 1978.

26. Gasset AR, Houde WL, Garcia-Bengochea M: Hard contact lens wear as an environmental risk in keratoconus, *Am J Ophthalmol* 85:339-341, 1978.

27. Macsai MS, Varley GA, Krachmer JH: Development of keratoconus after contact lens wear: patient characteristics, *Arch Ophthalmol* 108:534-538, 1990.

28. Mandell RB: Keratoconus. In: Mandell RB: *Contact Lens Practice,* 4th ed, Springfield, 1988, Charles C. Thomas, 824-849.

29. Swann PG, Waldron HE: Keratoconus: the clinical spectrum, *J Am Optom Assoc* 57:204-209, 1986.

30. Maguire LJ, Bourne WM: Corneal topography of early keratoconus, *Am J Ophthalmol* 108:107-112, 1989.

31. Mandell RB, Shie C: Validity of videokeratography [abstract], *Optom Vis Sci* 70(10):21, 1993.

32. Mandell RB, Polse KA: Keratoconus: spatial variation of corneal thickness as a diagnostic test, *Arch Ophthalmol* 82:182-188, 1969.
33. Edmund C: Corneal apex in keratoconic patients, *Am J Optom Physiol Opt* 64:905-908, 1987.
34. Korb DR, Finnemore VM, Herman JP: Apical changes and scarring in keratoconus as related to contact lens fitting techniques, *J Am Optom Assoc* 53:199-205, 1982.
35. Mackman GS, Polack FM, Sydrys L: Hurricane keratitis in penetrating keratoplasty, *Cornea* 2:31-34, 1983.
36. Kuwabara T, Perkins DG, Cogan DG: Sliding of the epithelium in experimental corneal wounds, *Inv Ophthalmol* 15:4-14, 1976.
37. Bron AJ: Vortex patterns of the corneal epithelium, *Trans Ophthalmol Soc UK* 93:455-472, 1973.
38. Fanta H. Acute keratoconus. In: Bellows JG, ed: *Contemporary Ophthalmology, Honoring Sir Stewart Duke-Elder,* Baltimore, 1972, Williams & Wilkins, 64-68.
39. Pierse D, Eustace P: Acute keratoconus in mongols, *Br J Ophthalmol* 55:50-54, 1971.
40. Caroline PJ, McGuire JR, Doughman DJ: Preliminary report on a new contact lens design for keratoconus, *Cont IOL Meds* 4:69-73, 1978.
41. Chiquiar-Arias V, Liberatore JC, Voss EH, Chiquiar-Arias M: A new technique of fitting contact lenses on keratoconus, *Contacto* 3:393-415, 1959.
42. Moss HI: The contour principle in corneal contact lens prescribing for keratoconus, *J Am Optom Assoc* 30:570-572, 1959.
43. Zadnik K, Mutti DO: Contact lens fitting relation and visual acuity in keratoconus, *Am J Optom Physiol Opt* 64:698-702, 1987.
44. Soper JW, Jarrett A: Results of a systematic approach to fitting keratoconus and corneal transplants, *Cont Lens Med Bull* 5:50-59, 1972.
45. Raber IM: Use of CAB Soper Cone contact lenses in keratoconus, *CLAO* 9:237-240, 1983.
46. Burger DS, Barr JT: Effects of contact lenses on keratoconus. In: Silbert JA: *Anterior Segment Complications of Contact Lens Wear,* New York, 1994, Churchill Livingstone, 379-399.
47. Caroline PJ, Doughman DJ, McGuire JR: A new contact lens design for keratoconus: a continuing report, *Cont Lens* 12:17-20, 1978.
48. Siviglia N: *The Ni-Cone keratoconus lens* [pamphlet], Lancaster, Pennsylvania, 1987, Lancaster Contact Lens, Inc.
49. Hartstein J: The correction of keratoconus with hydrophilic contact lenses, *Cont Lens Med Bull* 7:36-38, 1974.
50. Koliopoulos J, Tragakis M: Visual correction of keratoconus with soft contact lenses, *Ann Ophthalmol* 13:835-837, 1981.
51. Soper JW: Fitting keratoconus with piggy-back and Saturn II lenses, *Cont Lens Forum* 25-30, Aug 1986.
52. Woo GC, Callender MG, Egan DJ: Vision through corrected keratoconic eyes with two contact lens systems, *Int Cont Lens Clin* 11:748-756, 1984.
53. Caroline PJ, Doughman DJ: A new piggyback lens design for correction of irregular astigmatism: a preliminary report, *Cont Lens* 13:39-42, 1979.
54. Burger D, Bullimore MA, McMahon TT: Determining the nature of visual loss in keratoconus [abstract], *Optom Vis Sci* 67(10):96, 1990.
55. Herman JP: Flexure. In: Bennett ES, Grohe RM, eds: *Rigid Gas-Permeable Contact Lenses,* New York, 1986, Professional Press Books, 137-149.
56. Korb DR, Korb JE: A new concept in contact lens design: Parts I and II, *J Am Optom Assoc* 41:1023-1032, 1970.
57. Dietze TR, Durrie DS: Indications and treatment of keratoconus using epikeratophakia, *Ophthalmol* 95:236-246, 1988.
58. Boruchoff SA, Jensen AD, Dohlman CH: Comparison of suturing techniques in keratoplasty for keratoconus, *Ann Ophthalmol* 7:433-436, 1975.

59. Troutman RC, Gaster RN: Surgical advances and results of keratoconus, *Am J Ophthalmol* 90:131-136, 1980.
60. Paton RT, Swartz G: Keratoplasty for keratoconus, *Arch Ophthalmol* 61:370-372, 1959.
61. Richard JM, Paton D, Gasset AR: A comparison of penetrating keratoplasty and lamellar keratoplasty in the surgical management of keratoconus, *Am J Ophthalmol* 86:807-811, 1978.
62. Steinert RF, Wagoner MD: Long-term comparison of epikeratoplasty and penetrating keratoplasty for keratoconus, *Arch Ophthalmol* 106:493-496, 1988.
63. Gasset AR: Keratoconus, *Cont Lens Forum* 38-49, Jun 1977.
64. Itoi M, Nakaji Y, Nakae T: Keratoconus: the Japanese experience, *CLAO* 9:254-256, 1983.
65. Lembach RG, Lass JH, Stocker EG, Keates RH: The use of contact lenses after keratoconic epikeratoplasty, *Arch Ophthalmol* 107:364-368, 1989
66. McDonald MB, Safir A, Waring GO III, Schlichtemeier WR, Kissling GE, Kaufman HE: A preliminary comparative study of epikeratophakia or penetrating keratoplasty for keratoconus, *Am J Ophthalmol* 103(3 Pt 2):467, 1987.

Acknowledgment

The Medical Editing Department at Kaiser Foundation Research Institute provided editorial assistance for this chapter.

C H A P T E R

3

Therapeutic Soft Contact Lenses

Karla Zadnik

Key Terms

therapeutic contact lenses	soft contact lenses	corneal disease
bandage contact lenses	recurrent corneal erosion	

Many corneal conditions require correction with therapeutic soft contact lenses. These conditions all exhibit corneal epithelial compromise. The advent of hydrogel lenses revolutionized the ophthalmic practitioner's ability to enhance epithelial healing in eyes with mild (e.g., recurrent corneal erosions) to severe (e.g., alkali burns) corneal disease. Hydrogel contact lenses have applications as therapeutic bandages for damaged corneal epithelium. These lenses, as a therapeutic modality, require overnight wear for prolonged periods, sometimes weeks or months.[1] Unlike in conventional extended wear, patients do not typically handle these lenses themselves; indeed, one goal of bandage lens therapy is to disturb the epithelium as infrequently as possible.[1-3]

The following underlying mechanisms are common to most diagnoses requiring bandage lenses:[4]

1. Mechanical protection of the disrupted or healing epithelium from the environment (e.g., normal or abnormal lids or trichiatic lashes)

53

2. Structural reinforcement and promotion of vascularization of a weakened area of the cornea, such as a small perforation or a descemetocele
3. Relief from pain, especially in cases of bullous keratopathy

Indications

Indications for therapeutic lenses depend largely on the careful differential diagnosis of the corneal disease and a working knowledge of hydrogel contact lens use. Procedures unique to the prescribing of bandage lenses will be emphasized throughout this chapter.

Lens Types

The first therapeutic bandage lens that achieved wide use was the Bausch & Lomb Soflens Plano-T, a 38% water, ultrathin "membranous" lens.[4-8] This lens is still available, but medium and high water content lenses also are options now (Table 3-1). High water content lenses such as the Cooper Permalens are most useful for disorders in which the lens should cause as little trauma to the corneal epithelium as possible (e.g., bullous keratopathy, diffuse punctate epithelial keratopathy, and Thygeson's superficial punctate keratitis). Medium water content lenses (e.g., CIBA Softcon EW) are stiffer and are ideal for conditions in which the bandage lens functions as a splint or in which minimal lens movement is desirable. Conditions best treated

TABLE 3-1
Currently Approved Soft Contact Lenses for Therapeutic Use

Manufacturer	Material (percent water content)	Lens	Base curve/ series (mm)	Diameter
Bausch & Lomb	HEMA (38%)	Soflens	O3 O4	13.5 14.5
CIBA Vision	Vifilcon A (55%)	Softcon EW	7.8, 8.1, 8.4, 8.7 8.1, 8.4	14.0 14.5
CooperVision	Perfilcon A (71%)	Permalens	15.0 13.5 14.2	9.0 7.7, 8.0, 8.3 8.6
Lombart	Lidofilcon (79%)	LL-79	14.4	8.1, 8.4, 8.7
PBH	Crofilcon A (38.6%)	CSI Clarity Flexible Wear	13.8 14.8	8.0, 8.3, 8.6, 8.9 8.6, 8.9, 9.35

From White P, Scott C: Contact lenses and solution summary, *Cont Lens Spectrum Suppl,* 1994.

with this type of lens include wound dehiscence (separation of sutured wound margins), descemetocele (complete loss of stroma with only Descemet's membrane remaining), or small corneal perforation, and large nonhealing epithelial defects. There are specific advantages in fitting the medium water content lenses over the Permalens. For example, the Softcon lens comes in a variety of base curve and diameter parameters (Table 3-1), whereas the Permalens bandage lens has a 9.0 mm base curve and a 15.0 mm diameter; the other Permalens parameters are typically too small or steep for patients requiring bandage lenses. If the 9.0 mm to 15.0 mm lens does not fit the eye, high water content must be abandoned in favor of a larger variety of fitting parameters in the medium or low water content lenses. This same problem is encountered with the Bausch & Lomb Plano-T lens because it is manufactured in only one base curve and diameter, but the CSI lens (38% water), with more than one set of parameters, can be used.

CLINICAL PEARL

High water content lenses are most useful for disorders in which the lens should cause as little trauma to the corneal epithelium as possible. Medium water content lenses are stiffer and are ideal for conditions in which the bandage lens functions as a splint or in which minimal lens movement is desirable.

Additionally, investigators have reported on bandage lens case series using disposable hydrogel lenses.[9,10] These lenses certainly fulfill the oxygen delivery requirements of conventional soft bandage lenses. If they remain clean enough not to require too frequent manipulation, disposable lenses provide a viable means of contact lens therapy.

Postoperative Use

Many ocular surgical procedures can result in temporary epithelial disruption or frank epithelial defects. These include penetrating keratoplasty, epikeratoplasty, and vitrectomy in diabetic patients. Cataract extraction can be followed by corneal edema and bullous keratopathy. Most of these postsurgical conditions lend themselves well to bandage contact lens therapy.

In penetrating keratoplasty, lenses are most typically used for punctate epithelial keratopathy. "Hurricane" epithelial disruption has been described and associated with topical medication toxicity[11] and

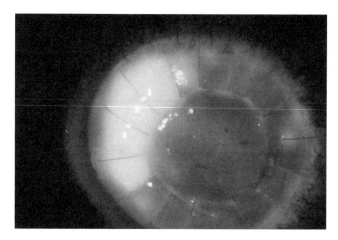

FIGURE 3-1 Intrasutural epithelial defect from recurrent *Acanthamoeba* keratitis after corneal transplantation.

appears clinically as punctate epithelial keratopathy. Any punctate epithelial keratopathy can be managed with bandage hydrogel lenses. Lenses are fitted to protect the epithelium from continued lid-induced trauma and to improve visual acuity by partially neutralizing any irregular astigmatism. As such, a nonmembranous lens with minimal movement is optimal.[12]

A postoperative persistent nonhealing epithelial defect following penetrating keratoplasty is most often seen in cases with preoperative diagnoses such as alkali burns, herpes zoster keratitis, dry eye, or *Acanthamoeba* keratitis (Figure 3-1). Treatment of these epithelial defects can include patching, but therapeutic contact lenses remain the therapy of choice. Some practitioners routinely fit bandage lenses immediately after surgery or at some prescribed time in the early postoperative period to promote epithelial healing and integrity and to protect the lids from sutural irritation.[13]

Another postoperative complication that is responsive to bandage soft contact lens therapy is early or late postoperative wound dehiscence. Mannis and Zadnik[14] report successfully repairing wound leaks in corneal transplant patients without surgical intervention by the application of medium water content, stiff, steep hydrogel lenses. The lenses promote vascularization at the donor-host interface in the dehiscence (Plate 9), and are often left in place for weeks or months to allow complete wound reapposition.

Epikeratoplasty is a surgical procedure now rarely used to correct myopia, aphakia, and keratoconus. It involves the suturing of a donor cornea lenticule into a keratectomy in the peripheral anterior stroma. Creation of a total epithelial defect in the host cornea underlying the onlay graft is vital to a successful surgical procedure. Typical postoperative instructions call for the application of a bandage contact lens either intraoperatively or immediately thereafter. Patients intolerant of bandage lenses are pressure patched. Therapeutic lenses are left in place, cycloplegic and antibiotic topical preparations are instilled, and the cornea reepithelializes.[15]

CLINICAL PEARL

In postoperative use, therapeutic lenses are left in place and concomitant cycloplegic and antibiotic topical preparations instilled until reepithelialization is complete.

Persistent epithelial defects are thought to occur in approximately 25% of diabetic patients after vitrectomy,[16] and therapy is similar to that for nonhealing epithelial defects in other conditions involving anesthetic and hypesthetic corneas. Arentsen and Tasman[17] reported on the prophylactic use of bandage contact lenses under the fundus during panretinal photocoagulation in diabetic patients to prevent incident corneal erosion.

Bullous keratopathy can occur after cataract surgery with intraocular lens implantation (pseudophakic bullous keratopathy, Plate 10), or without it (aphakic bullous keratopathy). Severe corneal edema results in the formation of epithelial bullae that can periodically rupture. Therapeutic lenses are known for their efficacy in relieving the pain associated with exposed nerve endings in bullous keratopathy (Table 3-2).[5-7,18,19] Their role in reversing the course of corneal edema

TABLE 3-2

Studies on Bandage Hydrogel Lens Use in Bullous Keratopathy

Author, Year	Sample Size (Number of Patients)	Study Type	Lens Type(s)	Pain Relief*	Visual Acuity†
Gasset and Kaufman, 1970[5]	12	Retrospective	Soflens, Bionite	++	++
Buxton and Locke, 1971[6]	6†	Prospective	Soflens	++	−−
Espy, 1971[19]	12	Prospective	Griffin	++	+
Hull et al, 1975[7]	29	Prospective but selected	Soflens	++	+
Hovding, 1984[18]	46	Prospective	Wohlk, Hydroflex 72	++	+
Smiddy, et al, 1990[1]	7	Retrospective	Permalens, Hydrocurve 55%	++	−−

*++, Good to excellent effect; +, Mild to good effect; −−, Poor to no effect.
†Hydrogel lenses were used in only one eye in each patient.

in terms of visual acuity and corneal thickness is less clear-cut. Hovding,[18] in a prospective study of hydrogel therapeutic contact lenses, found a modest but statistically significant improvement of one line in visual acuity in bullous keratopathy patients. This same study also demonstrated decreased corneal thickness after bandage lens application, but only when lenses were used in conjunction with topical hypertonic saline. Other studies used topical hypertonic saline without obvious positive or adverse effect.[5,6,19] Visual acuity improvement varied among investigators (see Table 3-2),[5-7,18,19] depending on the severity of corneal disease and the stiffness of the contact lens used. Espy's[19] use of the so-called Griffin lens, in particular, resulted in marked improvement in visual acuity. Resolution of corneal edema and improvement in visual acuity depend on whether the corneal edema is confined to the epithelium. Epithelial edema typically responds to hypertonic saline and the dehydrating effects of a hydrogel contact lens, and manifests irregular astigmatism that can be optically resurfaced by a contact lens.[5-7,18,19] In most cases of bullous keratopathy (especially advanced cases), therapeutic hydrogel lenses are used as a temporizing measure before further surgical intervention.

CLINICAL PEARL

Therapeutic lenses are known for their efficacy in relieving the pain associated with exposed nerve endings in bullous keratopathy. Their role in reversing the course of corneal edema in terms of visual acuity and corneal thickness is less clear-cut.

Epithelial Defects

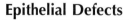

Epithelial defects occur in many shapes and sizes, from small recurrent erosions with minimal biomicroscopic evidence (Figure 3-2) to neurotrophic metaherpetic ulcers (Plate 11). Other epithelial defects are associated with stromal necrosis, as in the case of sterile ulcers, bacterial corneal ulcers, descemetoceles, and small corneal perforations. Therapeutic hydrogel lenses can assist in the management of these conditions.

Recurrent erosions are caused by a corneal dystrophy[20] or a previous episode of epithelial trauma, or are classified as idiopathic (see Figure 3-2). Within the corneal dystrophy category, the most common cause is epithelial basement membrane dystrophy (map-dot-fingerprint dystrophy or Cogan's microcystic dystrophy). Ten percent of these patients develop recurrent erosions, and fully 50% of patients presenting with recurrent erosions have been found to have epithelial basement membrane dystrophy.[21] Recurrent erosions also are associ-

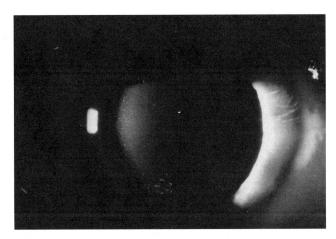

FIGURE 3-2 Epithelial dots characteristic of recurrent corneal erosion between acute episodes.

ated with Meesmann's juvenile epithelial dystrophy and Reis-Bücklers' ring-shaped dystrophy, two rare autosomal dominant diseases.[20]

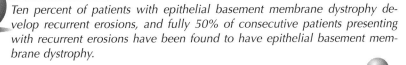

CLINICAL PEARL

Ten percent of patients with epithelial basement membrane dystrophy develop recurrent erosions, and fully 50% of consecutive patients presenting with recurrent erosions have been found to have epithelial basement membrane dystrophy.

Post-traumatic recurrent corneal erosions are most typically associated with a history of minor corneal injury from such agents as eye makeup applicators, fingernails or claws, branches, leaves, or paper edges.[4] Corneal erosions are thought to result from abnormal hemidesmosome attachments among the basal epithelium, epithelial basement membrane, and Bowman's layer, which regenerate during normal healing.[22] One group of investigators has reported that recurrent erosions caused by epithelial basement membrane dystrophy or prior trauma frequently occur in the inferior cornea, near the midline.[23]

Therapy for recurrent erosions runs the gamut from topical medications such as hypertonic saline solutions and ointments to shrink the epithelium and improve its adherence to the basement membrane[21] to bandage hydrogel contact lenses,[4] anterior stromal puncture,[24] or debridement.[21] Success rates as high as 100% with bandage lenses have been reported;[5] others achieve success in anywhere from

50% of patients[25] to 66% of eyes[26] and 70% to 80% of patients.[23,27] Williams and Buckley[28] randomly assigned 24 epithelial basement membrane dystrophy patients to treatment with hypertonic saline and ointment only or with therapeutic contact lenses and prophylactic topical antibiotics. These patients were compared to each other and to a group of traumatic recurrent erosion patients who were not randomized. Overall, patients treated only with topical preparations were less symptomatic as a group than the contact–lens-treated patients. Seven of the 11 contact lens wearers had complications other than recurrence of the original erosion. A retrospective study of 33 eyes of 25 recurrent erosion patients reported a 50% success rate for symptom relief, but patients with post-traumatic recurrent erosions or erosions from aphakic bullous keratopathy did worse with bandage lenses than did patients with epithelial basement membrane dystrophy or idiopathic erosions.[26]

The author's experience has been similar to that of Langston et al[26] in terms of success rates, but a differential response has not been noted according to the underlying cause of the erosion. Typically, a high water content large diameter lens with relatively flat base curve, or a medium water content, smaller diameter, slightly steeper lens is applied (see Table 3-1). Regardless of lens choice, as many patients experience alleviation of symptoms and healing of the eroded area as return the next morning with hyperemic, painful eyes requiring bandage lens removal. However, Mobilia and Foster[27] reported success with ultrathin lenses (CSI) and successfully fitted 12 patients with recurrent erosions who had previously failed with other types of hydrogel lenses. The major disadvantages of these lenses were difficulty with lens handling and frequent lens loss. Although therapeutic hydrogel lenses certainly have their place in the management of recurrent erosions, patients should be warned at the time of lens dispensing that the lens is by no means a panacea. It could be argued that a conservative 50% expected success rate should be presented to the patient.

Nonhealing epithelial defects associated with superficial sterile ulcers such as those seen in herpes simplex metaherpetic keratitis, neurotrophic ulcers in anesthetic or hypesthetic corneas (e.g., after neurological surgery or herpes zoster keratouveitis), or peripheral ulcers accompanying rheumatoid arthritis pose a particularly difficult task for the therapeutic hydrogel lens. In fact, these conditions respond well to bandage lenses. Eyes are not usually actively inflamed, so lenses are tolerated well. If left in place and not disturbed for several weeks (or occasionally months), complete epithelial healing with low rates of recurrent breakdown occurs.[16,19,24,28] One report of hydrophilic lens use in two patients with Mooren's ulcer showed dramatic pain relief without alteration of the disease's course.[29] In the case of peripheral ulcers the lens typically promotes desirable peripheral vascularization in the ulcerated area. Given this mechanism, the use of bandage lenses for central ulcers such as cylindrical ulcers in rheumatoid disease is a temporizing measure at best.

Lenses for these conditions should fit optimally, and a variety of lens types should be tried. Lenses should be manipulated as infrequently as possible. Typically, the epithelial defect's extent can be ascertained without instilling fluorescein, so lens removal for epithelial staining is unnecessary. These recommendations are unique to bandage lens application and do not apply to conventional cosmetic extended-wear lenses. Conventional extended wear requires weekly disinfection, and fluorescein-aided inspection of the corneal epithelium should be an integral part of routine follow-up care. The use of high molecular weight fluorescein is usually not more helpful than white light biomicroscopic viewing.

Corneal Perforations

The use of bandage hydrogels for impending or small corneal perforations can produce dramatic results. The use of bandage hydrogel lenses also has been reported for the long-term sealing of penetrating keratoplasty wounds,[8] and for descemetoceles,[30,31] perforations,[25] and even small corneal lacerations.[19,25,30,32]

In the case of descemetocele (Plate 12) (the anterior bulging of Descemet's membrane caused by intraocular pressure in an area devoid of stroma), corneal reinforcement can maintain a formed anterior chamber and prevent actual perforation.[30] Although one study reported that penetrating keratoplasty was performed 84% of the time as the primary therapy for descemetocele, hydrogel lenses were useful with or without cyanoacrylate glue in a small group of patients.[32] When surgery has to be delayed for some reason (for example, lack of donor tissue or the degree of ocular inflammation), a bandage lens can be an excellent temporizing measure, even for periods as long as 2 to 15 months.[30] Leibowitz and Berrospi[30] report success with the Bausch & Lomb Soflens, but current information advocates a stiffer, medium water content lens fitted with minimal movement to stent or split the distended tissue.[4,12,14]

Bandage lens application for corneal lacerations is specific to certain aspects of the wound.[33] It should be small (<3 mm)[4] and have well-apposed and aligned edges. Incarcerated uvea within the wound is a contraindication for bandage lenses. Advantages of this modality include no requirement for surgery, easy visualization of the wound's edges as healing occurs, rapid patient ambulation, and a resultant small, thin scar. Of course, the lens does not prevent invasive intervention if it becomes necessary.

In cases in which the corneal perforation or laceration is too large for spontaneous sealing to occur under a bandage soft contact lens and in which surgical repair is not desired, cyanoacrylate glue can be used. This results in an elevated, granular surface on the dried adhesive; bandage lenses have been used successfully to eliminate foreign body sensations and to prevent the glue from dislodging.[34,35]

Miscellaneous Conditions

Many rare conditions that chronically compromise the corneal epithelium can be treated with bandage hydrophilic lenses. These include lid-induced or lash-induced trauma in cases of entropion or trichiasis; bandage lenses provide a temporary cure before lid repair or cryoepilation.[26] Other conditions include primary ocular diseases such as Thygeson's superficial punctate keratitis, superior limbic keratitis, various dry eye conditions, cicatricial conjunctival disease,[5] alkali burns,[18] and acute hydrops in keratoconus.[6,18]

Thygeson's Superficial Punctate Keratitis

Thygeson's disease typically occurs in the third or fourth decade of life, and manifests as multiple, discrete epithelial lesions (Figure 3-3). It is usually a bilateral condition that has a chronic but intermittent course of as long as 7 years' duration. It is characterized by foreign body sensations that far outweigh the epithelial appearance, all in a white, quiet eye.[36-38] The symptoms are exquisitely sensitive to topical corticosteriods.[36-38] However, the ocular side effects of topical corticosteroids for chronic disease in young patients are considerable.

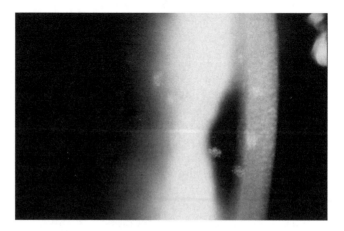

FIGURE 3-3 Epithelial lesions characteristic of Thygeson's superficial punctate keratitis.

Bandage lenses have been used successfully in the management of Thygeson's superficial keratitis. Both medium water content[39] and membrane type[40] lenses have been used in patients with long-term disease who demonstrate poor corticosteroid tolerance.

Superior Limbic Keratitis

Superior limbic keratitis is a chronic disease associated with tarsal and bulbar conjunctival inflammation superiorly, punctate staining of the superior cornea and limbus, and corneal filaments in approximately one third of patients. Therapy includes application of 0.5% silver nitrate solution to the superior tarsal conjunctiva and recession of the superior bulbar conjunctiva. Mondino et al[41] fitted six superior limbic keratitis patients with bandage lenses (type unspecified) in conjunction with pressure patching, resulting in elimination of the disease's signs and symptoms.

Dry Eye

As in routine hydrogel lens fitting, marginal dry eye or keratitis sicca is a relative contraindication to lens use. Early on, clinicians used bandage lenses in keratitis sicca and related dry eye conditions with good success. Most of these experiences were based on small numbers of patients and enthusiastic observers.[6,13,42] Since that time, however, reports of success with bandage lenses in dry eye patients have been few and far between, typically tempered by simultaneous reports of increased incidence of complications.[18,25] Hovding[18] advocates prophylactic topical antibiotics for dry eye patients wearing bandage lenses, but the author's experience is that dry eye patients do not tolerate the lenses well, except in severe cases with extreme pain. Lower water content lenses have been recommended for bandage lens use in dry eye patients.[3] In patients who require lenses, frequent use of artificial lubricants is mandated. One study has shown no accumulation of benzalkonium chloride in bandage lenses worn by dry eye patients,[43] but concerns about preservatives and pharmacological agents persist.[44]

Complications

Minor complications such as redness, irritation, and lens spoilage occur frequently with therapeutic hydrogel contact lens use. Tolerance and management of these complications differ from those of cosmetic hydrogel lens wearers because the potential benefits to the compromised cornea far outweigh the risks. The work of Dohlman et al[25] is the largest tabulation of complication rates in 278 bandage soft contact lens patients, and will be quoted in the statistics that follow (Table 3-3).

TABLE 3-3

Complications of Therapeutic Bandage Soft Contact Lenses in 278 Patients

Complication	Frequency	Percent
Lens not retained	35	12.5
Lens not tolerated	38	13.7
Deposits on lens	19	6.8
Neovascularization	8	2.9
Infiltrative keratitis	11	4.0
Severe infections	4	1.4

From Dohlman CH, Boruchoff SA, Mobilia EF: Complications in use of soft contact lenses in corneal disease, *Arch Ophthalmol* 90:367-371, 1973.

Injection and irritation may be transient or may result in discontinuation of lens wear. Corneal vascularization may actually be desirable in cases of sterile peripheral ulcers or penetrating keratoplasty wound leaks; it occurred in only 8 of 279 patients. Hovding[18] records it as his most common complication.

Infiltrative keratitis occurred in a small number of patients, with four patients contracting a severe corneal infection. More recently, a case series of 22 bandage contact-lens-associated corneal ulcers was reported. Bacterial keratitis occurred mostly in pseudophakic bullous keratopathy and neurotrophic keratitis patients. These cases were associated with gram-positive organisms and possible antibiotic or corticosteroid use.[45]

Use of Topical Agents

The potential for bacterial infection in a cornea with deranged epithelium suggests the advisability of prophylactic topical antibiotics for patients wearing therapeutic soft contact lenses. However, clinicians do not all agree that this is warranted in every situation or that it eliminates the risk of corneal ulcers. Binder and Worthen[46] found no change in the conjunctival flora of extended-wear soft contact lens wearers with application of various topical antibiotics. Dohlman et al[25] and other researchers[18,47] argue for the routine employment of topical antibiotics, whereas Nesburn[48] prescribes them during the first few days of therapeutic bandage lens wear, with eventual discontinuation.

The only absolute contraindication for topical antibiotic use during hydrogel lens wear is the use of epinephrine for intraocular pressure reduction. This particular compound discolors lenses and can result in corneal adrenochrome deposits.[48]

Some occurrences during therapeutic soft contact lens wear should not be classified as complications but simply represent a failure of the lens in its therapeutic role. These include the 50% of patients with unsuccessful recurrent erosion,[26] the bullous keratopathy patient with persistent bulla formation in spite of lens placement, and patients with nonhealing epithelial defects and descemetoceles that go on to perforate under the lens. Such events should not discourage the contact lens practitioner. In dealing with seriously diseased corneas, bandage soft contact lenses simply provide one method of management. Although they are not universally efficacious, they have rapidly become valuable tools in the contact lens armamentarium to manage the compromised corneal epithelium.

References

1. Smiddy WE, Hamburg TR, Kracher GP, Gottsch JD, Stark WJ: Therapeutic contact lenses, *Ophthalmol* 97:291-295, 1990.
2. Hayworth NA, Asbell PA: Therapeutic contact lenses, *CLAO* 16:291-295, 1990.
3. Plotnik RD, Mannis MJ, Schwab IR: Therapeutic contact lenses, *Int Ophthalmol Clin* 31:35-52, 1991.
4. McDermott ML, Chandler JW: Therapeutic uses of contact lenses, *Surv Ophthamol* 33:381-394, 1989.
5. Gasset AR, Kaufman HE: Therapeutic uses of hydrophilic contact lenses, *Am J Ophthalmol* 69:252-259, 1970.
6. Buxton JN, Locke CR: A therapeutic evaluation of hydrophilic contact lenses, *Am J Ophthalmol* 72:532-535, 1971.
7. Hull DS, Hyndiuk RA, Chin GN, Schultz RO: Clinical experience with the therapeutic hydrophilic contact lens, *Ann Ophthalmol* 7:555-562, 1975.
8. Levinson A, Weissman BA, Sachs U: Use of Bausch & Lomb Soflens plano T contact lens as a bandage, *Am J Optom Physiol Opt* 54:97-103, 1977.
9. Lindahl KJ, DePaolis MD, Aquavella JV, Temnycky GO, Erdey RA: Applications of hydrophilic disposable contact lenses as therapeutic bandages, *CLAO* 17:241-243, 1991.
10. Gruber E: The Acuvue disposable contact lens as a therapeutic bandage lens, *Ann Ophthalmol* 23:446-447, 1991.
11. Mackman GS, Polack FM, Sydrys L: Hurricane keratitis in penetrating keratoplasty, *Cornea* 2:31-34, 1983.
12. Zadnik K: Post-surgical contact lens alternatives, *Int Cont Lens Clin* 15:211-220, 1988.
13. Aquavella J, Shaw EL: Hydrophilic bandages in penetrating keratoplasty, *Ann Ophthalmol* 8:1207-1219, 1976.
14. Mannis MJ, Zadnik K: Hydrophilic contact lenses for wound stabilization in keratoplasty, *CLAO* 14:199-202, 1988.
15. McDonald MB, Kaufman HE, Durrie DS, Keates RH, Sanders DR: Epikeratophakia for keratoconus: The nationwide study, *Arch Ophthalmol* 104:1294-1300, 1986.
16. Mandelcorn MS, Blankenship G, Machemer R: Pars plana vitrectomy for the management of severe diabetic retinopathy, *Am J Ophthalmol* 81:561-570, 1976.
17. Arentsen JJ, Tasman W: Using a bandage contact lens to prevent recurrent corneal erosion during photocoagulation in patients with diabetes, *Am J Ophthalmol* 92:714-716, 1981.
18. Hovding G: Hydrophilic contact lenses in corneal disorders, *Acta Ophthalmol* 62:566-576, 1984.
19. Espy JW: Management of corneal problems with hydrophilic contact lenses, *Am J Ophthalmol* 72:521-526, 1971.
20. Waring GO, Rodrigues MM, Laibson PR: Corneal dystrophies. I. Dystrophies of the epithelium, Bowman's layer and stroma, *Surv Ophthalmol* 23:71-122, 1978.

21. Brown N, Bron A: Recurrent erosion of the cornea, *Br J Ophthalmol* 60:84-96, 1976.
22. Khodadoust AA, Silverstein AM, Kenyon KR, Dowling JR: Adhesion of regenerating corneal epithelium: the role of basement membrane, *Am J Ophthalmol* 65:339-348, 1968.
23. Hykin PG, Foss AE, Pavesio C, Dart JK: The natural history and management of recurrent corneal erosion: a prospective randomised trial, *Eye* 8:35-40, 1994.
24. McLean EN, MacRae SM, Rich LF: Recurrent erosion. Treatment by anterior stromal puncture, *Ophthalmol* 93:784-799, 1986.
25. Dohlman CH, Boruchoff SA, Mobilia EF: Complications in use of soft contact lenses in corneal disease, *Arch Ophthalmol* 90:367-371, 1973.
26. Langston RHS, Machamer CJ, Norman CW: Soft lens therapy for recurrent erosion syndrome, *Cont IOL Med J* 10:875-878, 1978.
27. Mobilia EF, Foster CS: The management of recurrent corneal erosions with ultra-thin lenses, *Cont IOL Med J* 4:25-29, 1978.
28. Williams R, Buckley RJ: Pathogenesis and treatment of recurrent erosion, *Br J Ophthalmol* 69:435-437, 1985.
29. Leibowitz HM, Rosenthal P: Hydrophilic contact lenses in corneal disease. I. Superficial, sterile, indolent ulcers, *Arch Ophthalmol* 85:163-166, 1971.
30. Leibowitz HM, Berropsi AR: Initial treatment of descemetocele with hydrophilic contact lenses, *Ann Ophthalmol* 7:1161-1166, 1975.
31. Joondeph HC, McCarthy WL, Rabb M, Constantaras AA: Mooren's ulcer: Two cases occurring after cataract extraction and treated with hydrophilic lens, *Ann Ophthalmol* 7:1161-1166, 1976.
32. Arentsen JJ, Laibson PR, Cohen EJ: Management of corneal descemetoceles and perforations, *Trans Am Ophthalmol Soc* 82:92-105, 1974.
33. Leibowitz HM: Hydrophilic contact lenses in corneal disease. IV. Penetrating corneal wounds, *Ann Ophthalmol* 88:602-606, 1972.
34. Hirst LW, Smiddy WE, Stark WJ: Corneal perforations. Changing methods of treatment 1960-1980, *Ophthalmol* 89:630-634, 1982.
35. Weiss JL, Williams P, Lindstrom RL, Doughman DJ: The use of tissue adhesives in corneal perforations, *Ophthalmol* 90:610-615, 1983.
36. Tantum LA: Superficial punctate keratitis of Thygeson, *J Am Optom Assoc* 53:985-986, 1982.
37. Thygeson P: Superficial punctate keratitis, *JAMA* 114:1544-1549, 1950.
38. Thygeson P: Further observations on superficial punctate keratitis, *Am J Ophthalmol* 66:158-162, 1961.
39. Forstot SL, Binder PS: Treatment of Thygeson's superficial punctate keratopathy [sic] with soft contact lenses, *Am J Ophthalmol* 88:186-189, 1979.
40. Goldberg DB, Schanzlin DJ, Brown SI: Management of Thygeson's superficial punctate keratitis, *Am J Ophthalmol* 89:22-24, 1980.
41. Mondino BJ, Zaidman GW, Salamon W: Use of pressure patching and soft contact lenses in superior limbic keratoconjunctivitis, *Arch Ophthalmol* 100:1932-1934, 1982.
42. Gasset AR, Kaufman HE: Hydrophilic lens therapy of severe keratitis sicca and conjunctival scarring, *Am J Ophthalmol* 71:1185-1189, 1971.
43. Lemp MA: Bandage lenses and the use of topical solutions containing preservatives, *Ann Ophthalmol* 10:1319-1321, 1978.
44. White P, Scott C: Contact lenses and solutions summary, *Cont Lens Spectrum* 1994.
45. Kent HD, Cohen EJ, Laibson PR, Arentsen JJ: Microbial keratitis and corneal ulceration associated with therapeutic soft contact lenses, *CLAO* 16:49-52, 1990.
46. Binder PS, Worthen DM: A continuous-wear hydrophilic lens: Prophylactic topical antibiotics, *Arch Ophthalmol* 94:2109-2111, 1976.
47. Thoft RA, Mobilia EF: Complications with therapeutic extended wear soft contact lenses, *Int Ophthalmol Clin* 21:197-208, 1981.
48. Nesburn AB: Complications associated with therapeutic soft contact lenses, *Ophthalmol* 86:1130-1137, 1979

4

Contact Lens Applications in Aphakia

Barry A. Weissman

Key Terms

cataract extraction	contact lenses	hydrogels
aphakia	rigid gas-permeable	

Cataract, the opacification of the intraocular crystalline lens, is a leading cause of blindness worldwide.[1] One recent study estimates that each year 20 million people (almost 4 million in India alone) develop visually disabling cataracts.[2,3] Many factors contribute to cataract's progression including metabolic disease (e.g., diabetes); uveitis; atopic dermatitis; familial inheritance; nutritional deficiencies and disorders; drugs (e.g., steroids); radiation; infrared, ultraviolet (UV) and perhaps even visible light;[4] and trauma. Age-dependent (or "senile") cataract is the most common form[5] (Figure 4-1).

Cataracts interfere with vision to varying degrees, depending on their development, density, and location within the crystalline lens (Figure 4-2). No proven medical treatments exist for cataract, although ultraviolet-filtering spectacles may act prophylactically. Surgical intervention is indicated when a cataract interferes with activities important or essential to the patient.

Cataract surgery is one of the most ancient and still one of the most common forms of surgery. Anecdotal reports suggest couching was practiced by the ancient Egyptians and Hindus. Daviel first formally

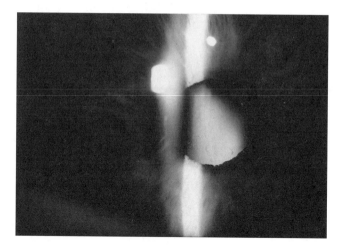

FIGURE 4-1 Cataract with vacuoles in the eye of a 65-year-old male patient.

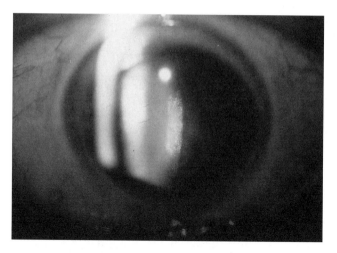

FIGURE 4-2 Posterior subcapsular cataract in the eye of a 60-year-old patient. This is more visually disabling than cataract in other areas of the lens.

proposed extracapsular extraction of the cataractous lens (ECCE) in 1748; Sharp introduced intracapsular cataract extraction (ICCE) shortly thereafter. The popularity of each approach has waxed and waned over the last two centuries because of complications and other contributing factors. A British ophthalmologist, Harold Ridley, implanted the first plastic polymethylmethacrylate (PMMA) intraocular lens (IOL) in 1949.[6] With major improvements in technology, experience, and skill providing improved results, the popularity of combined ECCE and intraocular lens implantation has increased over the last decade. The trend in the West is toward capsulectomy, ECCE by phacoemulsification, and smaller incisions (requiring few if any sutures) with foldable IOLs. ICCE, however, continues to be a common form of surgery in underdeveloped countries.[7]

The number of cataract extractions performed in the United States has grown from about 600,000 in 1983[8] to 1.5 million operations in 1992 and 1993, at an estimated cost to the American public of $50 billion for the decade 1983-1992.[9] More than 95% of patients from whom cataracts are extracted in this country receive IOLs (or "pseudophakia") in exchange.[10] These pseudophakia are usually posterior chamber IOLs. For the remaining 5% of aphakic eyes, optical correction is usually best achieved through contact lenses, and only secondarily by spectacles. This is more than a cosmetic decision. Contact lenses (like IOLs) usually produce vision similar to that experienced by the patient before the changes in his or her crystalline lens, as opposed to the magnified and distorted vision experienced with aphakic spectacles.[11,12] Epikeratophakia was proposed as another form of optical rehabilitation following cataract extraction, but failed to gain popularity.

CLINICAL PEARL

The number of cataract extractions performed in the United States has grown from about 600,000 in 1983 to 1.5 million operations in 1992 and 1993, at an estimated cost to the American public of $50 billion for the decade 1983-1992.

Optical Correction

The human eye has approximately 60 diopters of optical power, two thirds of which are contributed by the cornea, with most of the remainder being contributed by the crystalline lens. Following removal of the crystalline lens, the patient generally becomes hypermetropic. The exact refractive correction, however, depends on the final corneal curvature, which may have changed because of the surgery, and the eye's axial length. The final refraction also bears some relationship to the presurgical refractive error. For example, a patient who was severely myopic preoperatively might become only slightly hyperopic after surgery. Most patients, however, require more than +10 D in refractive correction after cataract extraction;[13] Benton and Welsh[14] found that 75% of cataract patients required between +11.75 D and +13.50 D correction in the spectacle plane. This leads to a relative image magnification of about 30%,[11,12] varying with the power needed and the vertex distance of the correcting lens. This magnification makes objects appear larger and closer. Variable magnification across the field of view leads to distortion. The use of aphakic spectacle lenses results in limited fields of vision. Aphakic patients whose vision is corrected with spectacles also experience a peripheral ring scotoma (called "jack in the box" because of the manner in which objects disappear and then reappear as they cross through visual space) related to the decrease in field of view; the prismatic effects of these strong glasses inhibit the patient's ability to see a portion of visual space around the lens' edge.[15,16]

If a patient has only one usable and aphakic eye, or is bilaterally aphakic, spectacle correction becomes an option. Many patients will accommodate and adjust to aphakic vision with spectacles, although few will like it.[17] Some patients (especially those with preexisting macular diseases) may experience improved central visual acuity because of the magnification of high plus-powered spectacles. The majority, however, will complain bitterly about changes in visual perception and report difficulties in walking, negotiating steps, pouring liquids, and driving motor vehicles.

Patients with unilateral aphakia (i.e., having a normal phakic fellow eye) are usually unable to adjust to the differences in magnification and distortion between the two eyes if spectacles are used for optical correction.[11] The difference in image size between the two eyes is too great for fusion to occur. Before the advent of contact lenses, in fact, good vision in the fellow eye was considered a relative contraindication to cataract extraction.

Contact lenses, like IOLs, decrease relative magnification. Magnification has been calculated to be between 5% and 10% when aphakia is corrected with contact lenses,[11,12] depending upon the exact circumstances. Although this level of magnification may initially cause some difficulties, the vast majority of patients are able to tolerate it.[18] To minimize anisometropia during the correction of unilateral aphakia, it is best to try to achieve isocorrection[12] (in other words, either maintain a similarly powered forward spectacle correction for each eye or fully correct both eyes with contact lenses). Isocorrection also means that the patient will not encounter prismatic difficulties when looking through spectacles in directions other than forward.

Contraindications for IOLs

There are still situations in which an IOL is not indicated. Because patients having these contraindicated conditions will become the pool of potential aphakic contact lens wearers, it is worth a few lines to discuss them. One contraindication is the patient's age.[19] Although the short-term safety and efficacy of IOLs is obvious from their clinical success, it is difficult to predict how long a patient will tolerate any foreign body within the eye. We have 20 years of data on various IOL designs, some that caused severe problems and have been abandoned,[20] and some that have been extremely successful. Thus a 60-year-old patient could reasonably expect to maintain problem-free useful vision for the remainder of his or her life following ECCE with implantation of a posterior chamber IOL. However, even the best current IOLs may eventually cause difficulties. Some surgeons are therefore reluctant to implant IOLs in patients younger than about 40 years. Very young children also occasionally develop cataracts from a number of etiologies (that will be discussed later). Most pediatric ophthalmologists feel IOLs are impractical in this setting because of optical power changes anticipated with ocular growth and because of fear about the device's morbidity within the eye over a child's lifetime.[21]

Intraocular disease, especially severe or recurrent uveitis, or abnormal anatomy (including aniridia or compromise to the iris or corneal endothelium) are other contraindications to use of IOLs.[22] Trauma may be severe enough to disorganize the eye's anterior segment, to damage the structures that would be needed to physically support an IOL, and to injure the corneal endothelium.

Diabetes, especially to the point where retinopathy is proliferative, has in the past been a contraindication for an iris-fixed IOL because of the attending clinician's need to observe the peripheral retina from time to time. Many diabetic patients, however, now successfully use posterior chamber IOLs.

Implantation in the presence of concurrent glaucoma or in a patient with only one usable eye is controversial. Glaucoma may compromise corneal endothelial cells, and rubeosis increases the risk of hemorrhage. The use of steroids to control inflammation either immediately after surgery or subsequently may complicate glaucoma therapy. Anterior chamber IOLs are contraindicated because of possible additional mechanical compromise of the angle, but posterior chamber IOLs are being used more frequently even by conservative practitioners. Similarly, some surgeons believe one-eyed patients are at risk and are reluctant to use an IOL in this setting. Other surgeons are now convinced that the risks of IOL implantation have decreased over the last several years so much that the obvious benefits of pseudophakic vision far outweigh the slight risk of additional complications.

An unplanned event during the surgical procedure itself may cause the operating surgeon to abandon the effort to implant an IOL. Such events produce another small group of patients who will be aphakic and in need of optical correction.

Finally, for a few very highly myopic patients an IOL is unnecessary because only minimal refractive correction will be required after simple cataract extraction.

Contact lens correction of aphakia therefore retains a clinical role despite the vast reduction in potential patients from those available several years ago.

Postsurgical Problems

Complications of cataract extraction are numerous and may affect the course of contact lens care. It is unnecessary to review all the possible complications of the surgical procedure, but it is appropriate to discuss important and pertinent potential problems. These complications can be divided into early and late difficulties and are rarely seen in isolation; most exist in a setting of shared etiologies and associations. Serious complications of cataract extraction often require immediate and aggressive medical or surgical management to minimize vision loss.

Complications Encountered in the Immediate Postoperative Period

Lid edema and ptosis from the trauma of the operative procedure may disturb the patient from a cosmetic viewpoint and also induce potential contact lens centration problems, especially with rigid contact lenses. Lid edema and postoperative ptosis, however, should at least partially resolve by the time the patient has healed sufficiently for contact lens fitting. Conjunctival hemorrhage, injection, anterior chamber flare, cells, and hyphema are not uncommon. Corneal edema (even with folds in Descement's membrane) from intraoperative trauma, damage to the corneal endothelium, or elevated intraocular pressure may be seen.

Pain is usually minimal; deep ocular pain should alert the clinician to consider corneal abrasion, elevated intraocular pressure, or infection.

Vitreous may occasionally be seen ballooning forward through the pupil into the anterior chamber following cataract extraction, especially ICCE. This is a particularly ominous sign, suggesting that the patient is at risk for pupillary block glaucoma, retinal detachments, cystoid macular edema, and endothelial decompensation if the vitreous should adhere to the cornea's posterior surface.[19]

Wound leak may be detected by a positive Seidel's sign during the prefitting or postfitting evaluations. Wound leaks may cause hypotonia, flattened anterior chambers, and choroidal detachments, and may invite endophthalmitis (vitreous wick syndrome). Shallowing of the anterior chamber, ocular hypotonia, and iris prolapse should alert the clinician to the possibility of this complication, but can occur without frank dehiscence of the surgical wound (e.g., ocular hypotonia can be secondary to choroidal detachment). Aphakic pupillary block is another potential cause of a flat anterior chamber in the early postoperative period, but intraocular pressure will be elevated, not reduced, in such an instance.

Hemorrhages are another possible complication of cataract extraction, either from the operative wound, the iris or ciliary body, or other areas. Trauma and defective wound healing may play a role. Intraocular hemorrhage may occur in the vitreous or lead to hyphema in the anterior chamber. Expulsive hemorrhage is a rare and disastrous event, but usually only occurs at the time of surgery.[23]

Many types of iris damage can occur during cataract extraction (including cyclodialysis clefts, iris tears and atrophy, and synechiae), occasionally resulting in enlarged and irregular pupils (Figure 4-3).

Some iritis or uveitis is common in the immediate post–cataract-extraction period, and may persist afterward to complicate the continued care of patients, especially those with concurrent glaucoma.

Jaffe wrote that infectious endophthalmitis was a rare and declining complication of cataract extraction in the early 1980s, occurring with an incidence of 0.35%.[19] Data gleaned from Medicare files suggests that this rate decreased from 0.12% in 1984 to 0.08% in beneficiaries operated upon in 1986 and 1987.[24] The patient's own conjunctiva and eyelids are the most likely source of infecting organisms in postoperative endophthalmitis.[25,26]

After surgery, however, wound leak, unplanned filtering blebs, suture abscess, and incarceration of iris (iris prolapse) or vitreous into the

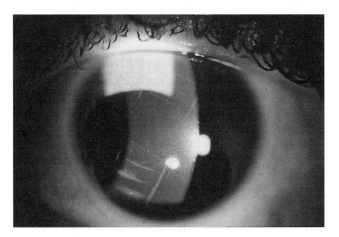

FIGURE 4-3 Anterior segment of the right eye of a 25-year-old female. This patient underwent radial keratotomy including astigmatic incisions approximately 18 months previously, and subsequently suffered an apparently unrelated retinal detachment (RD). Complications during the surgical repair of the RD left the patient aphakic and with an inferior defect in her iris.

wound are all potential risk factors for endophthalmitis. Contact lens wear is an additional risk.[27] Symptoms of intraocular inflammation (e.g., pain, hyperemia, conjunctival chemosis, lid edema, and anterior chamber and vitreous reactions, including hypopyon) should alert the clinician to possible endophthalmitis and the need for prompt aggressive management.

Glaucoma

Glaucoma is the end result of many of cataract surgery's complications. It may occur early or late, and according to Jaffe[19] is responsible for the largest number of eyes lost after cataract surgery. Specific etiologies include peripheral anterior synechiae formation resulting from delayed reforming of the anterior chamber, pupillary block,[28] phacoanaphylaxis, fibrous ingrowth or epithelial downgrowth, hyphema, and anterior and posterior chamber hemorrhage (more common in diabetic patients). Additional etiologies include prolonged intraocular inflammation, "UGH" syndrome (the combination of uveitis, glaucoma, and hyphema), and steroid response.

Potential Late Complications Associated with Cataract Extraction

The late complications of cataract extraction are important because they are commonly encountered during contact lens treatment of aphakic eyes. They often occur with the patient presenting during or after the contact lens fitting process with the observation that vision has diminished. The patient is usually not in pain or alarmed and symptoms are vague if a problem is noted at all. He or she often feels that the difficulty is lens related, resulting from change in power or difficulty in getting the lens clean. The clinician, after finding that the lens is performing well, must then distinguish among a set of possible problems in relatively white, quiet eyes.

Corneal edema and aphakic bullous keratopathy are among the more serious complications of cataract surgery.[19] The proposed etiology is that operative trauma following previous disease (e.g., uveitis, glaucoma, and Fuchs' dystrophy) has weakened the endothelium and reduced its ability to function with additional insult or normal aging. Endothelial cell counts lower than about 1000 cells/mm^2 (normal counts would be 1500 cells/mm^2 to 2000 cells/mm^2 or greater) and increased irregularity of the endothelial cell mosaic, including increased polymorphism and polmegethism, indicate increased risk of such corneal decompensation. Contact lens wear may provide an additional mechanical or physiological stress to the already compromised endothelium.[29] Surgical trauma, even in the absence of preexisting endothelial disease, has occasionally been implicated in the etiology of corneal edema and aphakic bullous keratopathy. Prolapse of the vitreous, adherence to the endothelium (particularly in the center of the cornea), or postsurgical epithelial downgrowth have been discussed as alternative causes of aphakic bullous keratopathy.

A small number of patients may develop Brown-McLean syndrome, a nonvascularized peripheral corneal edema, usually secondary to ICCE and rarely seen with ECCE.[30,31] It does not appear to be affected by or to affect contact lens wear directly, or to interfere with vision, because the edema is peripheral.

Opacification of lenticular material left by accident or by design within the eye after cataract extraction is another common cause of postoperative visual decline. Residual capsular epithelium may proliferate after surgery, forming "Elschnig's pearls." It may accumulate in clusters or be uniformly distributed. Scarring from residual lens cortex left in the eye following surgery can form a ringlike structure. With ECCE, the posterior capsule may initially be thin and transparent, but may later distort or opacify. Many of these opacifications in the optical axis are now approached noninvasively with Nd:YAG laser capsulotomy if vision is disturbed. However, this procedure may increase the risk of subsequent retinal complications, breaks, and detachment.[32]

Cystoid macular edema (CME) typically occurs 1 to 3 months or longer following an uneventful ICCE.[33] Risk factors include diabetes and cardiovascular disorders such as hypertension, previous heart attack, or stroke. Vision may drop to 20/100. Examination of the fundus may show the characteristic honeycomb appearance of the macular area, but fluorescein angiography may be needed to confirm the diagnosis. Many believe this macular lesion results from intraocular inflammation or vitreous traction. The edema is transient, and usually good vision will eventually be restored, but medical management is often indicated. Persistent CME, especially if associated with vitreous traction, may prompt surgical vitreolysis or vitrectomy. Other macular changes (e.g., epiretinal membranes) may occur to locally compromise the retina.

Retinal detachment is known to follow cataract extraction, most commonly within the first 6 months following surgery. An early incidence value was 2%,[34] but more recent data suggest that the cumulative probability of detachment is 0.81% within 3 years of surgery (data from 1986 and 1987).[24] Retinal detachment has been associated with the loss or prolapse of vitreous during cataract extraction, but the exact pathogenesis is unclear.[19] Other predisposing factors include axial myopia; retinal lattice degeneration; holes, tears, or previous detachment in the fellow eye; surgical trauma; and relative youth. Presenile cataract extraction offers greater risk of retinal detachment. Retinal detachment will only reduce central vision if the macula is involved, so other symptoms (such as an increase in floaters, photopsia, the appearance of a visual haze or "veil," or

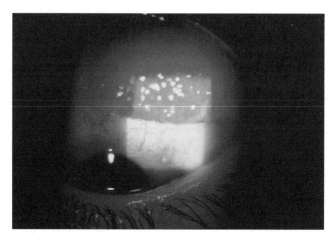

FIGURE 4-4 Suture-related giant papillary conjunctivitis (GPC) in the right eye of a 14-year-old girl 2 weeks after cataract extraction. The eliciting suture barb can be seen on the superior limbus.

sudden onset of distorted vision) should alert the clinician that thorough investigation is indicated.

Suture loosening or abscess and filtering blebs[27] also may be noted in the late postsurgical period, and may increase the risk of infectious endophthalmitis. Vision is usually unaffected, but loose sutures may cause discomfort and perhaps giant papillary conjunctivitis (GPC),[35] and also may serve as a locus for infection (Figure 4-4).

Clinical Evaluation

A patient presents with aphakia in one or both eyes. The clinican proceeds with a full evaluation of the patient's ophthalmic status (including baseline intraocular pressures and visual fields) directed toward visual rehabilitation. Several areas of concern are associated with aphakia, requiring more than a normal thorough examination.

While obtaining a complete history, the clinician should determine when, where, and by whom the cataracts were removed. What was the underlying etiology (if known)? Were there any intraoperative or postsurgical complications? Is there a history of ophthalmic surgery or disease (e.g., retinal detachment)? Does the patient have any history with contact lens wear, and does he or she have any predetermined perceptions?

It is probably best to wait 6 to 12 weeks after surgery before commencing contact lens fitting.[36] Stability of corneal curvature and refraction indicates the termination of the healing process; the clinician also should observe the wound and adnexa for signs of residual chemosis and inflammation. Very young children present a special situation because they heal much more rapidly than adults and require the optical correction of contact lenses for amblyopia much more rapidly. The author has successfully fitted and dispensed contact lenses to young children as soon as 1 or 2 weeks after surgery.

Corneal curvature is often modified by cataract extraction and secondary healing. It is not uncommon to find patients with substantial against-the-rule astigmatism[6] (associated with wound gape caused by loosening sutures), although microsurgery, improved suturing, and operating keratometers have decreased this problem's incidence and severity in recent years. Trauma or corneal grafting also can lead to irregular corneal surfaces. When astigmatism or irregularity is severe, corneal topography is often helpful in establishing which sutures should be removed or in selecting the initial contact lens approach. Even if only one eye is to be fitted with a lens, the clinician should measure the corneal curvature of both eyes so that comparisons may be made.

A careful refraction should be performed on both eyes. This allows the clinician to make a baseline assessment of the aphakic eye's expected visual acuity, modified by the exact situation. For example, one would anticipate Snellen vision with a contact lens to be slightly less improved than that with spectacle refraction in uncomplicated aphakia, because of magnification loss, but possibly improved over that attainable for a patient who lost his or her crystalline lens secondary to trauma that left the corneal surface scarred and irregular. Because it is best from a magnification standpoint to try to achieve isocorrection,[12] the clinician should know the fellow eye's refractive status. This will help the clinician decide whether to attempt full correction with a contact lens or leave the patient undercorrected or overcorrected so that forward spectacles will be of approximately equal optical power for both eyes.

During biomicroscopy, the clinician should examine the lid surfaces and margins, the cornea and the anterior segment, and the surgical wound. I find it helpful to count sutures and note their location on my chart. The clinician should check for loose or exposed sutures (which may be physically irritating, cause GPC, and encourage infection), wound dehiscence, planned or unplanned filtering blebs, and chemosis or inflammation. The pupil (which may be disfigured from surgery or trauma) should be examined and described, iridectomies noted, and the presence or absence of any pupillary membranes or posterior capsular remnants considered. Any scars or changes in the cornea such as Cogan's map-dot-fingerprint dystrophy (Figure 4-5), which is not uncommon among the elderly, should be described, and any anterior synechiae, endothelial guttae, or corneal endothelial precipitates noted.

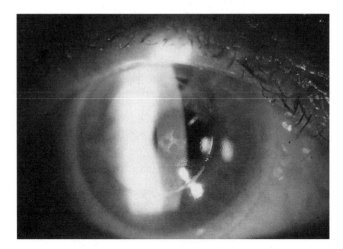

FIGURE 4-5. Anterior basement membrane dystrophy (Cogan's map-dot-fingerprint) is seen beneath a hydrogel contact lens worn successfully on the aphakic right eye of a 70-year-old woman.

Mechanical Problems

The primary mechanical problem in aphakic contact lens application is obtaining adequate lens centration. This can be because of the physical construction of high plus-powered contact lenses with thick centers and thin edges. These lenses tend to position inferiorly because of the combination of advanced center of gravity, increased overall weight, and tapered edges. Corneal surface irregularities; problems with lid structure, tension, and dynamics; and the interaction of these factors also combine to make lens centration difficult.

Lens Construction

A plus-powered contact lens may be manufactured with a single curve or with many curves on its front surface. All current hydrogel contact lenses known to the author use bicurve, minus-carrier, or lenticular, anterior construction. Rigid lenses are manufactured in lenticular design or, alternately, in large or small diameter "single-cut" designs[37,38] (Figure 4-6).

Lenticular lenses offer improved centration, all things being equal, by decreasing weight,[39] by changing the position of the lens' center of gravity, and by providing the upper lid with a minus-powered design edge.[40] Large single-cut plus-powered lenses tend to position low on the cornea and become immobile. Therefore if the patient has relatively steep corneal curvature with minimal astigmatism, a small

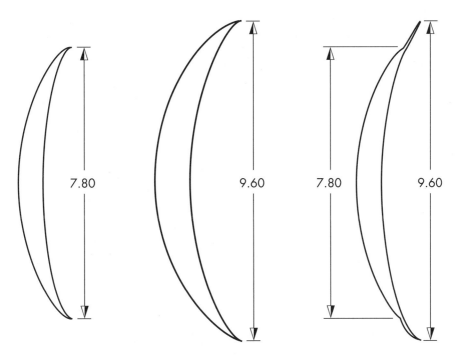

FIGURE 4-6 Cross-sectional profiles of high plus-powered contact lens designs. All lenses are intended to be +15.00 diopters in power and of 7.70 mm base curve. The far left design is single-cut and of small (7.8 mm) overall diameter. The middle design is single-cut but of larger (9.6 mm) overall diameter. The far right design is a lenticular lens profile with an overall diameter of 9.6 mm, but with an anterior optical cap diameter of 7.8 mm. All three lens designs show a single posterior peripheral curve of 10.0 mm radius and 0.3 mm width. Central thicknesses are *left* 0.299 mm, *middle* 0.501 mm, and *right* 0.398 mm. (Courtesy Richard Weisbarth, OD, Ciba Vision Corporation, Atlanta, Georgia.)

single-cut rigid lens may suffice to achieve good centration, movement, and tear exchange.[37] These small single-cut lenses allow good vision if pupil size and shape are not compromised, and usually maintain corneal physiology through their mobility and tear exchange. Polymethylmethacrylate (PMMA) opticap lenses were successful alternatives to the large single-cut lens until the introduction of rigid gas-permeable (RGP) plastics. Most clinicians today, however, restrict their primary lens designs to lenticular RGPs and hydrogels, although there may be times when single-cut rigid designs (either large or small-thin) of gas-permeable or impermeable materials might have specific value.

CLINICAL PEARL

Lenticular lenses offer improved centration, all things being equal, by decreasing weight, by changing the position of the lens' center of gravity, and by providing the upper lid with a minus-powered design edge.

Special Aspects of Rigid Lens Care

Compared to hydrogels, rigid contact lenses offer the aphakic patient good vision and ease of care. However, rigid lenses are less comfortable than hydrogels for a majority of patients, and this major problem restricts their use.

It is best to fit most eyes with large overall diameter (about 9.4 mm to 9.6 mm) lenticular RGP designs. The clinician should select an initial diagnostic lens with a base curve radius close to the flat K reading (0.25 DK to 0.50 DK flatter than K if corneal curvatures are relatively spherical, and 0.50 DK to 1.00 DK steeper than K if substantially astigmatic). The clinical goal is to determine a base curve radius that will result in light central corneal alignment or touch at a diameter that allows slightly high centration and under-the-upper-lid ride. This will distribute the lens' weight over the broadest possible epithelial area, allow tear exchange, and minimize 3 to 9 o'clock stain (believed to be more associated with low-riding than with high-riding RGP lenses). The clinician can achieve this goal through manipulation of overall diameter, front optic cap diameter, base curve radius, and peripheral curve construction. If corneal curvature is relatively steep (46.00 D or greater) and spherical, a small single-cut lens becomes an option (Figure 4-7).

Alternatively, some clinicians employ the opticap design. Opticap lenses can be fitted on central or slightly steeper alignment to achieve centration because the small overall diameters (about 8.0 mm) reduce lens weight, encourage tear exchange, and cover only a small portion of the corneal surface. Centration is critical, however, because of the limited optical zones of these small opticap lenses.

Large single-cut designs should be avoided except if the need exists to make a lens drop into a more inferior corneal position, or when duplicating a lens for a patient adapted to a certain lens design and intolerant of any other.

Rigid contact lenses should be manufactured from one of the various gas-permeable plastics. Evidence is overwhelming that corneal respiration must be maintained for a contact lens to be tolerated over the long term.[41]

Against-the-rule corneal astigmatism is a major mechanical barrier to successful rigid lens application following cataract extraction. In

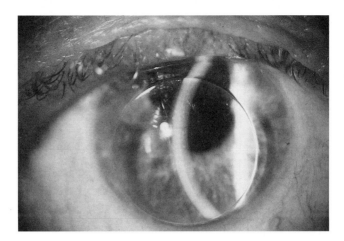

FIGURE 4-7 A small opticap single-cut design rigid polymethyl-methacrylate (PMMA) contact lens on the aphakic right eye of a geriatric patient. Note the lens' slightly inferior position and "keyhole" pupil. This patient showed slight 3 to 9 o'clock stain, but no corneal edema (CCC or ECF) was noted. Vision was 20/25.

many instances the astigmatism has been generated by the surgical procedure itself.[19] Against-the-rule corneal astigmatism induces rigid lens decentration (primarily laterally and secondarily inferiorly). Lens decentration can compromise vision, produce physiological complications, and decrease comfort. Decentration may occasionally be overcome through reduced optical cap diameter, lenticular constructions, and larger than normal lens diameters. In other instances, however, it is best to use a combined lenticularization and spherical power effect bitoric design.[42] A final option is to discontinue rigid lens wear and use a larger hydrogel contact lens that will center better; however, the patient will then require forward astigmatic spectacles and may not even then attain full visual potential.

Corneal irregularity is rare with modern uncomplicated cataract extraction. However, because of the IOL's popularity with the majority of surgical patients, many aphakic patients referred for contact lenses have additional complicating factors (such as previous ocular trauma and corneal grafts) that lead to irregular corneal topography. These patients should be addressed principally with rigid contact lenses because the chief goal is usually visual. It is easier to obtain good vision with a rigid lens than with a hydrogel lens. Keratometric curvature measurements and corneal topography assist in selection of initial base curve, somewhere between mean and flat K. Overall lens diameters are usually large, about 9.4 mm or greater. Diagnostic evaluation allows observation of centration, movement, and lens alignment with the corneal surface, aiding adjustment of lens fit.

Overrefraction establishes optical power requirement. The clinical goal is to select a contact lens with a base curve, diameter, and peripheral curve at the proper power for maximum vision, that will move and center adequately and be tolerable to the patient. The ideal lens also should show a fluorescein pattern with one third of the lens surface in alignment with the anterior corneal surface and two thirds pooling while maintaining good tear exchange during the blink. If astigmatism is somewhat regular, a spherical power effect bitoric design may be appropriate.[42] Hydrogel lenses may be employed if it proves impossible to attain these goals with various rigid lens designs (including bitorics and lenticularization). However, visual acuity may not be optimal with a hydrogel, even if corrected with forward astigmatic spectacles, because of corneal irregularity and variable vision.

One fairly common occurrence in the author's experience is the asymptomatic aphakic patient with 20 years of contact lens wear who presents for a progress evaluation successfully wearing a low-riding, large diameter, single-cut PMMA contact lens. Substantial corneal edema, circular clouding,[43] microcystic edema, or edematous formations[44] may be seen in the inferior cornea (Plate 13). The clinician must discuss this situation with the patient, and with the documented observation of corneal edema must advise refitting the patient with RGP lenses. The first choice lens material should be a mid Dk value (about 30×10^{-9} cm^2 ml O$_2$ sec ml mm Hg) in lenticular design, to improve centration and tear exchange while increasing the lens material's permeability. Optics are usually easily obtained, but many patients react to the higher riding lenticular lens with a strong foreign body sensation. Improvement in corneal sensation because of the resumption of proper oxygen supply[45] will only add to this problem as the corneal edema resolves. If this difficulty proves insurmountable, the patient should be returned to a low-riding single-cut design made from a highly oxygen-permeable material (i.e., Dk value greater than 40×10^{-9}). This lens will be quite thick, and the patient's progress should be followed closely.

In another common clinical situation, aphakic patients with a long history of PMMA lens wear present with no corneal edema or other problems. The author takes a conservative approach here. If there is no evidence of corneal edema or other difficulties, the clinician should discuss and document the need for RGP lenses with the patient, but should not initiate a refit unless the patient requests it.

Hydrogel Contact Lenses

The primary reason for using a hydrogel contact lens to correct optical aphakia is discomfort with RGP lens use. A second indication is the inability to attain adequate centration with RGP application. Hydrogel lenses are more difficult to maintain, more fragile, and give poorer visual results depending on the amount and regularity of any astigmatism, corneal irregularity, or tear deficiency. Substantial refractive (primarily corneal) astigmatism, corneal irregularity, and relatively poor tear layers are the major contraindications to the use of hydrogels. The clinician must consider the advantages and disadvantages in each clinical situation; in many cases indications and contraindications coexist.

Modern high plus-powered hydrogel contact lenses are all of lenticular design (although at one time they may have been single-cut),[46] and the vast majority of patient corneal topographies are approachable with the proper selection of lens base curve and diameter. Disposable or frequent replacement hydrogel lenses are not yet available in high enough powers for most aphakic patients. The author prefers to use low water content (nonionic) daily-wear hydrogel lenses that can be heat sterilized, but these are provided by few manufacturers. If difficulties in maintaining clean lens surfaces are encountered or if a high-water content or ionic material is needed, peroxide sterilization rather than heat sterilization is suggested. Appropriate enzyme use is extremely helpful (Table 4-1).

Hydrogel lenses are usually simple to insert. The initial lens is roughly 14.0 mm in diameter with a base curve radius about 1 mm flatter than the mean corneal curvature. Clinical observation after equilibration suggests changes in base curve radius or diameter to provide a lens that will center reasonably well on the ocular surface and move gently upon digital pressure. Many aphakic patients are elderly and have flaccid lids; their hydrogel lenses do not move well with simple blinking. Appropriate optical power is determined by retinoscopy and subjective refraction with diagnostic lenses in position on the eye.

Parameter variability is made possible by use of several brands and knowledge of what each laboratory will supply. Small diameter optic caps are acceptable for patients with little astigmatism whose pupils are round and normal and whose lenses center well. If some corneal irregularity or astigmatism must be optically masked, or if the patient has abnormally large pupils, it is advantageous to use hydrogel lenses with relatively large optic caps. Such lenses seem to mask more of the astigmatism (both regular and irregular), and can improve attainable visual acuity. Some concern must be expressed, however, about the potential decrease in oxygen transmissibility with large optic caps and centrally thick designs in low water content plastics. Complications caused by hypoxia with these lenses have been rare in the author's practice, but both stromal swelling and corneal vascularization have occasionally been noted (Plate 14). Perhaps the relatively thin periphery of these lenses allows enough oxygen to reach the underlying tear film so that minimal (and perhaps reduced compared to the needs of

TABLE 4-1

Manufacturers of Aphakic Hydrogel Contact Lenses and Their Available Parameters

Manufacturer/ Lens Name Size	Base Curve/Overall Diameter (mm)	Water Content/Type (%$H_2$0/Chemistry)	Vertex Power (Measured)	Optic Cap Size (mm)
Ocular Sciences/				
Hydron Mini	8.1 to 8.9/13.0	38/nonionic	back	8.0
Bausch & Lomb/				
Soflens N	8.3/12.5	38/nonionic	back	7.8
F3	8.4/13.5	38/nonionic	back	7.8
H3	8.3/13.5	38/nonionic	back	9.0
H4	8.8/14.5	38/nonionic	back	9.0
CW 79*	8.1 to 8.8/14.4	79/nonionic	back	8.0
Ciba/Sofcon*	7.8 to 8.7/14 to 14.5	55/ionic	back	7.5
Cooper-Coastvision				
Hydrasoft*†	8.3 to 8.9/14.2 to 15	55/ionic	front	8.4
Permalens*	8.0 to 8.9/14 to 14.5	71/ionic	back	6.4 to 7.9
Kontur				
Kontur 55†	8.3 to 8.9/15	55/ionic	front	6.5 to 8.0
Metro Optics				
Metrosoft	8.6 to 8.9/13.5	38/nonionic	front	9.0
Wesley-Jessen				
Durasoft 2	8.2 to 8.5/13.5	38/ionic	back	8.0
	8.3 to 9.0/14.5	38/ionic	back	8.0
3*	8.3 to 9.0/14.5	55/ionic	back	8.0

From Contact lens Index. *J Am Optom Assoc.* 60:240, 1989; Tyler's Quarterly Soft Contact lens Parameter Guide, *Quarterly Tyler's Publication,* Little Rock, ARK, December 1988; Lowther GE: Updated lens classification tables. *Int Cont Lens Clin* 15:205, 1988; General Ophthalmics: *Tori-Check Guide.* General Ophthalmics, Inc, Park Ridge, IL, 1987. * Indicates FDA approved for extended wear; † Indicates available in > +20 D power.

the phakic population)[47-49] corneal oxygen requirements are met for most patients.

Depressed tear production in the elderly aphakic population is a particularly vexing problem for both patient and clinician. Hypothetically, a high water content, high plus-powered contact lens may lose up to 2.5 D of optical power with dehydration;[50] the author has clinically observed one patient decrease to −2 D in such a setting. Inadequate tears also make the lens less tolerable over the long term, resulting in surfaces that dry out and become less effective, and that soil and age rapidly. Changes in comfort (possibly secondary to base curve, diameter variability, and surface drying) may be induced as well. Patients with particularly poor tear layers should wear RGP lenses if at all possible.

Problems of the Geriatric Aphakic Patient

Most aphakic individuals are elderly and many have tear layer abnormalities including epiphora and depressed tear volume (espe-

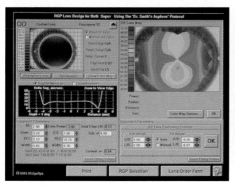

PLATE 1

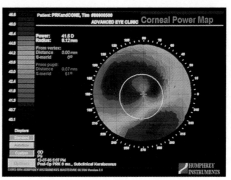

PLATE 2

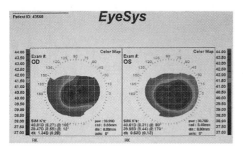

PLATE 3

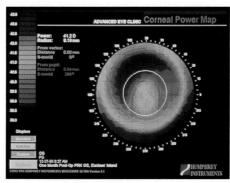

PLATE 4

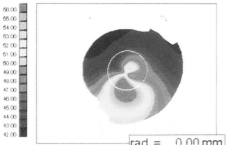

PLATE 5

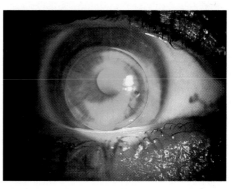

PLATE 6

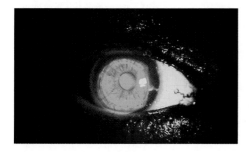

PLATE 7

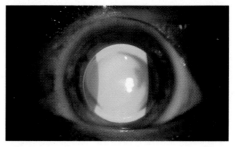

PLATE 8

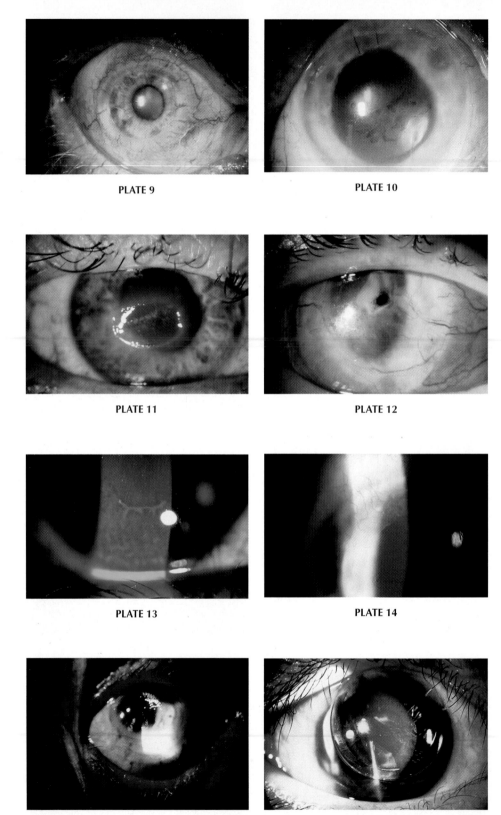

PLATE 9

PLATE 10

PLATE 11

PLATE 12

PLATE 13

PLATE 14

PLATE 15

PLATE 16

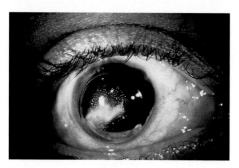

PLATE 17

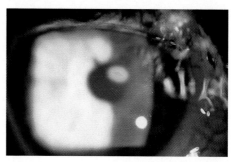

PLATE 18

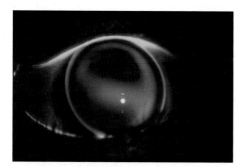

PLATE 19 (A)

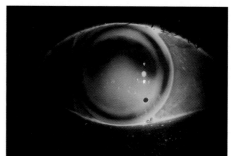

PLATE 19 (B)

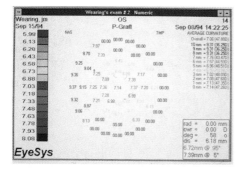

PLATE 20 (A)

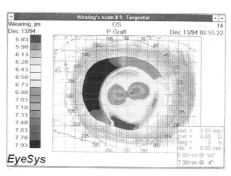

PLATE 20 (B)

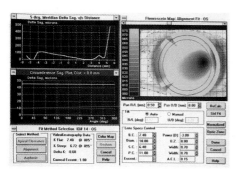

PLATE 20 (C)

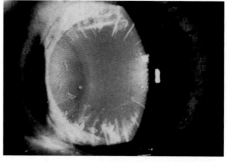

PLATE 21

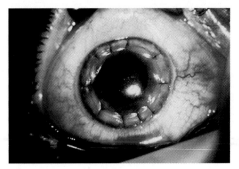

PLATE 22

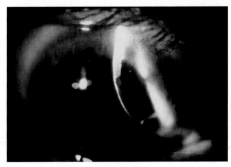

PLATE 23

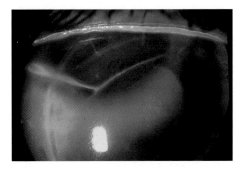

PLATE 24

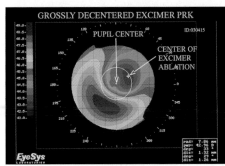

PLATE 25

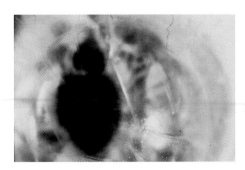

PLATE 26 (A)

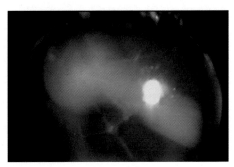

PLATE 26 (B)

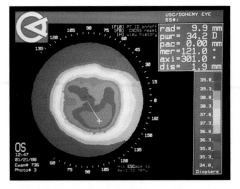

PLATE 27 (A)

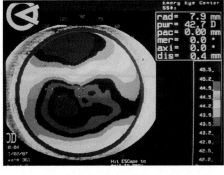

PLATE 27 (B)

PLATE 1 Simulated fluorescein pattern in combination with the patient's color map. (Courtesy EyeSys.)

PLATE 2 Patient appears to have subclinical keratoconus but underwent PRK and is now seen at 6 months postoperatively. (Courtesy Humphrey Instruments.)

PLATE 3 Patient, in Plate 2, has central flattening and midperipheral steepening, characteristic of post-radial keratotomy. (Courtesy EyeSys.)

PLATE 4 Examination shows a very subtle excimer laser–induced central island located over the visual axis 1 month after PRK. (Courtesy Humphrey Instruments.)

PLATE 5 Map of keratoconic cornea. (Courtesy EyeSys.)

PLATE 6 Tight contact lens.

PLATE 7 Lens imprint on cornea.

PLATE 8 Modified contact lens.

PLATE 9 Wound vascularization after wound dehiscence promoted by application of a hydrogel bandage lens.

PLATE 10 Pseudophakic bullous keratopathy.

PLATE 11 Neurotrophic corneal ulcer associated with herpes zoster ophthalmicus.

PLATE 12 Central, small descemetocele in dry eye accompanying rheumatoid arthritis.

PLATE 13 Edematous corneal formation (ECF) is seen in the inferior right cornea of a 25-year-old man. This patient had congenital cataracts removed 20 years previously and successfully wore large diameter single-cut design rigid polymethylmethacrylate (PMMA) contact lenses. These lenses positioned inferiorly with poor movement, but with excellent vision (20/25) and tolerance. The patient was successfully refitted into lenticular construction RGPs to the same vision, and the ECF resolved over 6 months.

PLATE 14 Substantial superficial corneal neovascularization in the superior right cornea of a 70-year-old bilaterally aphakic man who wore hydrogel contact lenses and occasionally napped with the lenses on his eyes.

PLATE 15 Severely soiled high water content hydrogel contact lens on the aphakic right eye of a 75-year-old woman. Note the hard white deposits in the lens and inferior superfical neovascularization in the cornea, both secondary to extended wear.

PLATE 16 Rigid gas-permeable lenticular design high plus–powered contact lens on the aphakic eye of an 8-year-old child after traumatic injury. Note vertical trauma scar in the inferior cornea.

PLATE 17 Rigid gas-permeable lenticular design high plus–powered contact lens on an adult man's aphakic eye; the cataract in this case was secondary to penetrating trauma. Note the larger scar in the inferior cornea and the almost total loss of iris. Also note the bubbles under the lens from corneal irregularity leading to dimple veil staining.

PLATE 18 Oval full-thickness epithelial defect in the right cornea of a 70-year-old woman wearing a rigid gas-permeable lens for correction of unilateral aphakia with 20/20 vision. Symptoms were minimal on presentation for a routine progress evaluation 5 years after fitting.

PLATE 19 **A,** Against-the-rule proud graft fitted with an OK85 lens. **B,** Superiorly tilted proud graft fitted with an OK85 lens.

PLATE 20 **A,** EyeSys tangential plot of a proud, with-the-rule graft showing a flat nasal host. **B,** Numeric (keratometric) data of the same eye. The large curvature change from the graft-to-host margin on the nasal side is striking. C, Simulated fluorescein pattern of an OK85 lens and the tear layer thickness between lens and eye. (Courtesy EyeSys.)

PLATE 21 Sato placed his incisions on the cornea's posterior side to flatten the front surface. Although it took some time to occur in the Asian population, corneal decompensation resulted.

PLATE 22 Although performed on a limited basis, epikeratoplasty can provide tectonic support and temporary corneal flattening in the patient with keratoconus.

PLATE 23 Intrastromal hematoma (hemorrhage) is shown after contact lens wear in a patient with radial keratotomy.

PLATE 24 Unfortunately, in this case the wrong axis was identified as the steepest meridian, and a Ruiz procedure had to be performed 90 degrees from the initial radial incisions.

PLATE 25 Decentered ablation area. This often results in astigmatism and reduced best-corrected spectacle acuity. (Courtesy EyeSys.)

PLATE 26 **A** and **B**, Fluorescein patterns show areas of zonal bearing (*dark band*) when a lens has been applied.

PLATE 27 **A**, Dioptric map of a patient with radial keratotomy. The warmer colors show an area of steepening. Cooler colors reflect central corneal flattening. **B**, Multifocal effect helps explain acceptable distance and near vision in a 50-year-old patient with radial keratotomy.

cially among women). Their lids may demonstrate entropion, ectropion, poor functional action, and a decrease in tension. Chronic blepharitis, meibomian gland dysfunction, and lagophthalmos may further compromise lid and tear function.

Elderly patients have other diseases. Some of these, such as diabetes, chronic blepharitis, Sjögren's syndrome (dry eye, dry mouth, and arthritis with lymphocytic infiltration of the lacrimal gland suggesting an autoimmune etiology), and acne rosacea suggest that these patients are more prone to develop dry eyes, epithelial erosion, corneal vascularization, and infection while using contact lenses. Other diseases simply complicate their lives, giving them a variety of medications to obtain, maintain, and use, in addition to the complicated care systems with which the contact lens clinician tries to inspire compliance. Some of these medications also may depress tear supply.

Lid hygiene, tear supplements, medical treatment of lid disorders, and blinking exercises may all assist in contact lens application, but these chronic problems are rarely easily, completely, or conclusively addressed.

Elderly patients frequently are less dexterous and trainable at lens care procedures than their younger counterparts. Lens loss and damage may become an emotional and financial burden. Near vision is usually compromised, making lens care even more difficult.

Yet many elderly patients, given patience and conscientious instruction, will do amazingly well at learning contact lens care. The elderly aphakic patient is often motivated, and corneal oxygen requirements, swelling response, and sensitivity may be suppressed[47-49] and reduced by aging and the preceding surgery. Additionally, a subgroup exists for whom a friend or spouse may serve as lens care provider.

Extended or Daily Wear?

If any contact lens wearers could benefit from extended wear, it would seem to be elderly aphakic patients. Unfortunately, the initial enthusiasm for hydrogel extended wear[51-53] has been tempered by the increased occurrence of infection,[54,55] acute red eye reactions, corneal vascularization, and giant papillary conjunctivitis (GPC) in both phakic and aphakic patient populations.[51-59] The author believes that the incidence of these complications in the elderly aphakic population was blunted by a concomitant rise in IOL use. Elderly aphakic patients are probably still being fitted with hydrogel lenses for extended-wear use, but the numbers are declining and hopefully caution is being exercised.

Extended wear is only an option of last resort for the aphakic population; daily wear should be used whenever possible because of the increased risks associated with extended wear. For extended-wear patients, the clinical choice is a high water content (to promote oxygenation), FDA-approved extended-wear hydrogel contact lens.

The patient should be fully instructed in lens care and perhaps assisted by a friend or relative. The patient should remove the contact lens once or twice a week, clean it with both surfactant and appropriate enzyme, and sterilize it with a minimum 1 hour soak in a 3% hydrogen peroxide contact lens disinfecting solution. Peroxide neutralization should be completed before reinsertion. The patient should sleep without the lens and reinsert it, when cleaned, in the morning.[62]

CLINICAL PEARL

Extended wear is only an option of last resort for the aphakic population; daily wear should be used whenever possible because of the increased risks associated with extended wear.

The patient also should be instructed to be alert for signs of problems, especially infection. Infection usually presents as a foreign body sensation that increases and becomes painful; the eye then becomes red and discharge occurs.[63] The patient becomes photophobic. At the earliest moment the patient should remove the lens and return to the practitioner's care or seek immediate emergency care. Prompt professional attention and aggressive antibiotic therapy (without steroids or patching) is vital for the preservation of vision.

Even in the absence of any difficulties, the extended-wear patient should be reexamined at 3-month intervals (Plate 15). It has been suggested that replacing even a usable lens at these regular visits is a good method to reduce the incidence of GPC, acute red eye, and infection.[64]

RGP lenses have been used for extended wear in the aphakic group with mixed results.[65-67] The FDA, however, has not approved the manufacture of rigid lens materials otherwise approved for extended wear in powers greater than +12 D, effectively excluding the bulk of the aphakic population.

Children

Cataract is rare in children, but far from unknown. It has been estimated that between 10% and 40% of all visual impairment in children is caused by cataracts, and that the incidence of lenticular opacity in infants is close to 0.5%; etiologies are numerous.[68] A common diagnosis is persistent hyperplastic primary vitreous (PHPV), but clinicians also will provide care for babies with familial cataracts or with cataracts secondary to diseases such as in-utero rubella, uveitis (associated with juvenile rheumatoid arthritis), and

trauma. Pike et al[69] classified the etiologies of bilateral cataracts in 97 children into the following groups:
1. Heredity (23%)
2. Syndromes and metabolic disorders (9%)
3. Congenital infection (36%)
4. Trauma (1%)
5. Unknown (31%)

CLINICAL PEARL

It has been estimated that between 10% and 40% of all visual impairment in children is caused by cataracts, and that the incidence of leticular opacity in infants is close to 0.5%; etiologies are numerous.

Aphakic children benefit from contact lenses. Both academics and ophthalmic clinicians believe that aggressive contact lens care and amblyopia therapy offer the best possibility for the unilaterally aphakic child to optimize that eye's visual development. Bilaterally aphakic children do well with spectacle correction, but perhaps function more normally with contact lenses.

All types of contact lens modalities have been proposed, including rigid, hydrogel (soft), and flexible silicone. However, it is best to use hydrogels for very young children (younger than 6 months old) because it is easier for parents to handle and psychologically accept these lenses. Such lenses are usually (but not universally) custom manufactured, steep in base curve (8.00 mm or steeper) and high in power (+30 diopters or more). Although a small diameter lens (13.0 mm) should initially be prescribed to allow easy insertion, by the time the child is 2 months old a larger diameter (15.0 mm) semiscleral design will usually be required to prevent rapid lens loss. Retinoscopy over high plus-powered trial contact lenses defines needed power, decreasing difficulties from the effects of vertex distance. It is best to be somewhat over plus-powered to allow for near point fixation until the child begins to walk, at which time the lens power should be set for distance vision and additional near point correction provided. Any difficulties with astigmatism, corneal irregularity from trauma, or lens retention can be addressed with a rigid gas-permeable lens. Silicone elastomer lenses work best for children who are extremely uncooperative (usually 2-year-olds and 3-year-olds, following trauma), allowing parents to learn handling and care procedures on a durable contact lens. A rare extended-wear experience with these lenses should not be a problem. Daily-wear hydrogel (Figure 4-8) and RGP lenses (Plate 16) are usually employed with the standard care outlined previously, except that parents and guardians are responsible for care.

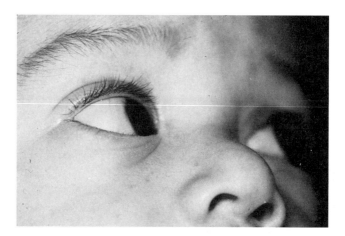

FIGURE 4-8 Bilateral hydrogel contact lenses on the eyes of a bilaterally aphakic 1-year-old boy.

Other authors[70,71] suggest extended wear for the pediatric group. However, it is rarely necessary, and concerns about complications (especially corneal infection and neovascularization) should lead the clinician to primarily prescribe daily wear.[72]

Complications with daily-wear contact lenses are minimal, including occasional slight (1 mm to 2 mm) superficial corneal vascularization (perhaps secondary to too much unplanned napping in daily-wear hydrogel lenses) and, rarely, abrasions from aggressive parental contact lens removal.

When followed aggressively, with much parental and professional attention and frequent lens changes to optimize optics and fit, aphakic children tolerate contact lenses well. A 1992 clinical study indicates the efficacy of contact lenses for aphakic pediatric patients. After cataract extraction, 111 children were referred from three pediatric ophthalmologists from 1980 to 1990. Clinical charts from these patients were reviewed, and 28 eyes were studied (14 from 7 bilaterally aphakic patients and 14 from unilaterally aphakic patients) for visual outcomes. Of the 14 bilaterally aphakic eyes, 11 (79%) had developed visual acuity of 20/40 or better, and three eyes (21%) developed vision between 20/40 and 20/200. Of the 14 unilateral cases, two eyes achieved vision of 20/40 or better, two eyes had vision between 20/40 and 20/200, and 10 eyes (71%) had vision worse than 20/200.[72]

Young Adults

The principal etiology of cataract development in young adults is ocular trauma. Less common etiologies include developmental or familial cataract, chronic uveitis (perhaps further complicated by steroid treatment), and atopic dermatitis. Subluxation from Marfan's syndrome also can lead the clinician to suggest a contact lens designed to provide vision through an aphakic portion of the visual axis in a young adult.

Application of contact lenses in the young adult group is identical to applications in the elderly, but the younger age group accepts lens care and handling more readily than the more senior group of patients. The younger age group also has less concomitant dry eye and other ocular and anterior segment abnormalities.

Intraocular trauma victims often have corneal scars and other cosmetic and mechanical disruptions of the normal anatomy of the eye's anterior segment. Fitting requires manipulation of rigid lens parameters (Plate 17), including occasional use of toric and bitoric rigid lenses to attain the best visual results. If vision is attainable, this should be the primary goal. Only if vision is limited or unattainable should cosmesis be a primary goal of contact lens fitting, because cosmetic work is difficult and expensive, and often precludes optimal visual correction.

Younger aphakic patients with iris defects are often bothered by glare. Pinhole rigid lenses may be prescribed, but most patients require artificial irides of about 11.0 mm diameter, larger than most RGP lens designs. Also, there is no FDA approval for painting RGP lenses, nor is it certain that the device's oxygen transmissibility is maintained if one or more surfaces is painted. Some custom hydrogel prostheses are available for such special cases in tints that act as density filters or with artificial irides (Figure 4-9)[73]; however, vision may not be optimal or cosmesis perfect in such situations.

A subgroup of patients with concomitant chronic uveitis deserves additional comment. These patients often show endothelial deposits that do not compromise vision but should be clinically monitored. The clinician must be alert to glaucoma indicated by pigment in the angle and inflammation. The condition may be a response to chronic steroid use. Steroids also depress immunological defenses and the patient's ability to resist infection. Patients who chronically use topical steroid drops should only be fitted with contact lenses if the clinical benefits outweigh the risk of corneal infection (aphakia is certainly such a condition). Fitting can proceed once the patient is fully apprised of the situation and agrees to the procedure (informed consent), and when the clinician trusts the patient to carefully maintain his or her contact lenses and solutions and to present for care at the first indication of complications.

Complications Associated with Contact Lens Wear

The complications associated with contact lens wear are generally the same regardless of age group or refractive error. Elderly aphakic patients as a group are more at risk for infection because hygiene may

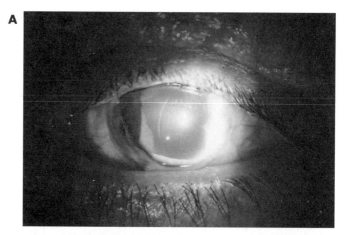

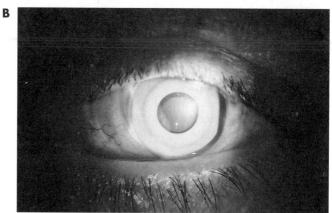

FIGURE 4-9 The left eye of a middle-aged man, aphakic secondary to blunt trauma. **A,** Note the significant loss of iris tissue. **B,** The eye wears a custom prosthetic hydrogel with artificial colored iris; optical power is +10 diopters. With this lens on the eye and forward astigmatic spectacle correction, the patient achieved 20/25 vision.

be less than stringent and because certain diseases such as diabetes[56] may make these patients less resistant. Extended wear appears to increase the incidence and severity of all complications known to occur with contact lens wear.[59-61]

Damage and soilage are probably the most commonly encountered complications of contact lens wear; virtually all patients will encounter problems in these areas if they wear lenses long enough (Plate 15). Giant papillary conjunctivitis (GPC) and incidents of acute red eye are associated with soiled or damaged lenses.[74-76]

Most other complications are associated with hypoxia, although modern oxygen-permeable rigid and hydrogel materials for daily wear minimize this group of complications. Biomicroscopy will note central corneal clouding (CCC)[43] in the epithelium following rigid (especially impermeable) contact lens wear. If chronic, CCC may induce wrinkling of the epithelial surface and produce edematous corneal formations (Plate 13).[44] Other forms of corneal edema from hypoxia are less easily observed. The epithelium may become edematous and show a microcystic appearance in retroillumination; similarly, epithelial microcysts may develop with extended wear.[76] Research has shown hypoxic epithelium to grow thin,[77] decrease in sensitivity[78] and mitosis,[79] and become less adhesive to underlying tissues.[80,81] The stroma also may grow thin.[77] The endothelium may develop blebs[82] and show chronic polymegethism.[83] Aphakic bullous keratopathy may result from poor endothelial function that has been additionally stressed by contact lens wear[29] or concomitant glaucoma.

Superficial corneal vascularization (Plate 14) also is a sequela of hypoxia with contact lens wear,[53,84-87] but is quite easily clinically monitored. The aphakic patient normally undergoes some vascularization of the incision wound; when covered by a contact lens these vessels may distend. If substantial distension is noted, the patient is usually sleeping or napping with the contact lens on the eye (even daily-wear lenses). This should be discouraged, not only to prevent vascularization but also to reduce the possibility of infection. Other, rarer etiologies for neovascularization include contact lens superior limbic keratoconjunctivitis (CLSLK), which has been associated with hydrogel lenses and thimerosal-preserved care solutions,[88] and vascularization of chronic 3 to 9 o'clock stain patterns. If daily wear is unsuccessful in stabilizing vascularization (especially if the vessels are stromal), an RGP lens of high Dk value will usually cause the vessels to become ghosts and not progress.

Epithelial staining is a generalized response to many etiologies. Patterns in the epithelium are helpful in diagnosis; 3 to 9 o'clock stain is usually caused by drying of the peripheral cornea at the edge of a rigid lens showing inferior displacement. This stain pattern also occurs if edge lift is too high, or indicates mechanical chafing if edge lift is insufficient. A central patch of stain may indicate a rigid contact lens over-wear abrasion. Occasionally epithelial defects develop apparently spontaneously (Plate 18). Staining of the inferior third of the cornea is most commonly caused by dry eye and lagophthalmos, and usually not by contact lens wear. Similarly, staining of the superior third of the cornea may be caused by superior limbic keratoconjunctivitis. Staining and infiltration at the corneal periphery, where the lids cross the limbus, may be caused by staphylococcal lid infections. Generalized stain may indicate viral infection or a chemical keratitis.

Solution sensitivities may produce many signs and symptoms. Generalized irritation associated with lens use may be eased by switching solutions. Generalized corneal stain or conjunctival injection may result from a toxic reaction.[89] Central infiltrates without epithelial defect,[90] epithelial pseudodendrites,[91] and contact–lens-associated SLK[88] have all been associated with thimerosal reactions. The clinician should be cautious in diagnosis; however, because similar signs may be noted with corneal diseases unrelated to contact lens wear.

If a corneal infiltrate is seen in association with an epithelial layer defect, the clinician must first suspect direct corneal infection. The presence of pain, photophobia, discharge, and anterior chamber reaction should heighten concern.[63] Microbial corneal infection is the most feared complication of contact lens wear. Infection is rare with daily wear and good care, but because most patients are noncompliant with good care[92] and often harbor potentially pathogenic microorganisms in some aspect of their care systems,[93] the clinician should always be on guard. Elderly patients tend to have suppressed immunity and more collateral diseases, and corneal sensitivity may be compromised somewhat by aging and the cataract extraction procedure; the clinician following the aphakic patient should be doubly on guard. About 0.1% of phakic patients using daily-wear lenses may develop a corneal infection. This is almost always in a setting of noncompliance, whereas about 1% of phakic and 2% of aphakic patients sleeping with contact lenses on their eyes (extended wear) may have a corneal infection even though some of these patients may be quite compliant.[94] Although the majority of infections in the contact–lens-wearing population are bacterial (principally culture positive for *Pseudomonas*), fungal infection appears more commonly in association with hydrogel extended wear in aphakic patients and therapeutic situations.[95] A potential corneal infection requires immediate and aggressive management and treatment.

Ultraviolet Filters

Mounting scientific evidence indicates that exposure to ultraviolet (UV) light may be a factor in various human diseases including skin cancer and some forms of cataract.[4] It also is likely that UV plays a role in some retinal diseases, particularly age-related macular degeneration.[96] Several RGP materials are now available with UV filtration; these should be used where appropriate for aphakic patients who have lost the normal filtration provided by the crystalline lens. Few hydrogel lenses are currently available with UV filtration and none specifically in aphakic powers, but it is hoped that manufacturers will begin to provide these lenses. Patients should continue to use supplemental UV-filtering spectacles for added protection.

Conclusion

Although their numbers are declining with the increasing success of IOLs, aphakic patients are among those who most benefit from the application of modern contact lenses. For those who are not able to have IOLs implanted, contact lens therapy is the best method to achieve visual rehabilitation. Advances in contact lens care over the last two decades have given these patients (through the hands of skilled and conscientious clinicians) devices of much improved safety and efficacy. Application in this group of patients requires time, patience, and care, but is emotionally rewarding to both clinician and patient when successful.

References

1. World Health Organization: Prevention of Blindness. Cataract—a major blinding condition, *Weekly Epidem Rec* 57:397, 1982.
2. Taylor HR, Sommer A: Cataract surgery: a global perspective, *Arch Ophthalmol* 108:797, 1990.
3. Minassian DC, Mehra V: 3.8 million blinded by cataract each year; projections from the first epidemiological study of the incidence of cataract blindness in India, *Br J Ophthalmol* 74:341, 1990.
4. Taylor HR, West SK, Rosenthal FS, Munoz B, Newland HS, Abbey H, Emmitt EA: Effect of ultraviolet radiation on cataract formation, *New Eng J Med* 319:1429, 1988.
5. Sasaki K, Hockwin O, Leske MC: *Cataract Epidemiology,* 1987, Karger, Basel.
6. Ridley H: The origin and objectives of intraocular lenticular implants, *Trans Am Acad Ophthalmol Oto* 81:OP65-OP67, 1976.
7. Agapitos PJ: Cataract surgery techniques, *Curr Opin Ophthalmol* 2:17, 1991.
8. Graves EJ: 1983 Summary: National Hospital Discharge Survey. Advance data from vital and health statistics, No 101; US Public Health Service Publication 84-1250. Hyattsville, Maryland, U.S. Public Health Service, 1984.
9. Young RW: Optometry and the preservation of visual health, *Optom Vis Sci* 70:255, 1993.
10. Jaffe NS, Jaffe MS, Jaffe GF: *Cataract Surgery and Its Complications,* St Louis, 1990, Mosby.
11. Ogle KN, Burian HM, Bannon RE: On the correction of unilateral aphakia with contact lenses, *Arch Ophthalmol* 59:639, 1958.
12. Craven PM, Smith G: Schematic eye predictions of relative spectacle magnification in unilateral aphakia, *Am J Optom Physiol Opt* 63:881, 1986.
13. Borish I: Aphakia: perceptual and refractive problems of spectacle correction, *J Am Optom Assoc* 54:701, 1983.
14. Benton CD, Welsh RC: *Spectacles for Aphakia,* Springfield, 1966, CC Thomas.
15. Dabezies O: Defects of vision through aphakic spectacles (part 1), *Cont Lens* 2:8-18, 1976.
16. Dabezies O: Defects of vision through aphakic spectacles (part 2), *Cont Lens* 2:8-20, 1976.
17. Anon (Woods AC): Adjustment to aphakia, *Am J Ophthalmol* 35:118-122, 1952.
18. Weis DR: Long-term results wearing hard contact lenses in monocular aphakia, *Ophthalmol* 89:1003, 1982.
19. Jaffe NS: *Cataract Surgery,* 4th ed., St. Louis, 1984, Mosby.
20. Mamalis N, Apple DJ, Brady SE, Notz RG, Olson RJ: Pathological and scanning electron microscope evaluation of the 91Z intraocular lens, *Am IOL Soc J* 10:191, 1984.
21. Neumann D, Weissman BA: Use of contact lenses in infants. In Isenberg S(ed): *The Eye in Infancy,* 2nd ed., St. Louis, 1994, Mosby.
22. Roper-Hall MJ: Intraocular lenses. In Duane TD(ed): *Clinical Ophthalmology Volume 5,* Philadelphia, 1983, Harper and Row.
23. Pau H: Der zeitfacktor bei der expulsiven blutung, *Klin Auggenheilkd* 132:865, 1958.
24. Javitt JC, Street DA, Tielsch JM et al: National outcomes of cataract extraction, *Ophthalmol* 101:100-105, 1994.

25. Leopold IH, Apt L: Postoperative intraocular infections, *Am J Ophthalmol* 50:1225-1247, 1960.
26. Speaker MG, Milch FA, Shah MK, Eisner W, Kreiswirth BN: Role of external bacterial flora in the pathogenesis of acute postoperative endophthalmitis, *Ophthalmol* 98:639-649, 1991.
27. Bellows AR, McCully JP: Endophthalmitis in aphakic patients with unplanned filtering blebs wearing contact lenses, *Ophthalmol* 88:839, 1981.
28. Sugar HS: Pupillary block and pupillary block glaucoma following cataract extraction, *Am J Ophthalmol* 61:435, 1966.
29. Nirankari VS, Baer JC: Persistent corneal edema in aphakic eyes from daily wear and extended wear contact lenses, *Am J Ophthalmol* 98:329, 1984.
30. Brown SI, McLean JM: Peripheral corneal edema after cataract extraction: a new clinical entity, *Trans Am Acad Ophthalmol Oto* 73:465, 1969.
31. Reed JW, Cain LR, Weaver RG, Oberfeld SM: Clinical and pathological findings of aphakic peripheral corneal edema: Brown-McLean Syndrome, *Cornea* 11:577, 1992.
32. Javitt JC, Tielsch JM, Canner JK, Kolb MM, Sommer A, Steinberg EP, and the Cataract Patient Outcomes Research Team: National outcomes of cataract extraction. Increased risk of retinal complications associated with Nd:YAG laser capsulotomy, *Ophthalmol* 99:1487-1497, 1992.
33. Gass JDM, Norton EWD: Cystoid macular edema and papilledema following cataract extraction: a fluorescein funduscopic and angiographic study, *Arch Ophthalmol* 76:646, 1966.
34. Shepland CD: Retinal detachment in aphakia, *Trans Ophthalmol Soc UK* 54:176, 1934.
35. Nirankari VS, Karesh JW, Richards RD: Complications of exposed monofilament sutures, *Am J Ophthalmol* 95:515, 1983.
36. Polse KA: Prefitting care of the aphakic patient, *Int Cont Lens Clin* 2:26, 1975.
37. Welsh RC: Corneal contact lenses trial sets for postoperative cataract patients, *Arch Ophthalmol* 65:427, 1961.
38. Polse KA: Hard lens aphakic fitting procedures, *Int Cont Lens Clin* 2:45, 1975.
39. Weissman BA: Mass of rigid contact lenses, *Am J Optom Physiol Opt* 62:322, 1985.
40. Nelson G, Mandell RB: The relationship between minus carrier design and performance, *Int Cont Lens Clin* 2:75, 1975.
41. Holden BA, Brennan NA, Efron N, Swarbrick HA: The contact lens: physiological considerations. In Aquavella JV, Rao GN (eds): *Contact Lenses,* Philadelphia, 1987, JP Lippincott.
42. Weissman BA, Chun MW: The use of spherical power effect bitoric rigid contact lenses in hospital practice, *J Am Optom Assoc* 58:626, 1987.
43. Korb DR, Exford JM: The phenomenon of central circular clouding, *J Am Optom Assoc* 39:223, 1968.
44. Korb DR: Edematous corneal formations, *J Am Optom Assoc* 44:246, 1973.
45. Bergenske PD, Polse KA: The effects of rigid gas permeable lenses on corneal sensitivity, *J Am Optom Assoc* 58:212, 1987.
46. Carter DB, Brucker D: Hydrophilic contact lenses for aphakia, *Am J Optom Arch Am Acad Optom* 50:316, 1973.
47. Korb DR, Richmond PP, and Herman JP: Physiological response of the cornea to hydrogel contact lenses before and after cataract extraction, *J Am Optom Assoc* 51:267, 1980.
48. Chaston J, Fatt I: Corneal oxygen uptake under a soft contact lens in phakic and aphakic eyes, *Inv Ophthalmol Vis Sci* 23:234, 1982.
49. Polse KA, Holden BA, Sweeney D: Corneal edema accompanying aphakic extended lens wear, *Arch Ophthalmol* 101:1038, 1983.
50. Fatt I, Chaston J: Swelling factors of hydrogels and the effect of deswelling (drying) in the eye on power of a soft contact lens, *Int Cont Lens Clin* 9:146, 1982.
51. Gasset AR, Lobo L, Houde W: Permanent wear of soft contact lenses in aphakic eyes, *Am J Ophthalmol* 83:115, 1977.

52. Stark WJ, Kracher GP, Cowan CL, Taylor HR, Hirst LW, Oyakawa RT: Extended wear contact lenses and intraocular lenses for aphakic correction, *Am J Ophthalmol* 88:535, 1979.

53. Mobilia EF, Foster CS: A comparison of various extended wear lenses for use in aphakia, *Contact and IOL Med J* 8:12, 1982.

54. Oxford Cataract Treatment and Evaluation Team: The use of contact lenses to correct aphakia in clinical trial of cataract management, *Eye* 4:138, 1990.

55. Glynn RJ, Schein OD, Seddon JM, Poggio EC, Goodfellow JR, Scardino VA, Shannon MJ, Kenyon KR: The incidence of ulcerative keratitis among aphakic contact lens wearers in New England, *Arch Ophthalmol* 109:104, 1991.

56. Eichenbaum JW, Feldstein M, Podos SM: Extended wear aphakic soft contact lenses and corneal ulcers, *Br J Ophthalmol* 66:663, 1982.

57. Spoor TC, Hartel WC, Wynn P, Spoor DK: Complications of continuous wear soft contact lenses in a non-referral population, *Arch Ophthalmol* 102: 1312, 1984.

58. Graham CM, Dart DKG, Buckely RJ: Extended wear hydrogel and daily wear hard contact lenses in aphakia, *Ophthalmol* 93:1489, 1986.

59. Weissman BA, Remba MJ, Fugedy E: Results of the extended wear contact lens survey of the Contact Lens Section of the AOA, *J Am Optom Assoc* 58:166, 1987.

60. Weissman BA, Mondino BJ, Pettit TH, Hofbauer JD: Corneal ulcers associated with extended wear soft contact lenses, *Am J Ophthalmol* 97:476, 1984.

61. Mondino BJ, Weissman BA, Farb MD, Pettit TH: Corneal ulcers associated with daily wear and extended wear contact lenses, *Am J Ophthalmol* 102: 58, 1986.

62. Kotow M, Grant T, Holden BA: Avoiding ocular complications during hydrogel extended wear, *Int Cont Lens Clin* 14:95, 1987.

63. Stein RM, Clinch TE, Cohen EJ, Genvert GI, Arentsen JJ, Laibson PR: Infected vs sterile corneal infiltrates in contact lens wearers, *Am J Ophthalmol* 105:632, 1988.

64. Kotow M, Holden BA, Grant T: The value of regular replacement of low water content contact lenses for extended wear, *J Am Optom Assoc* 58:461, 1987.

65. Welsh RC: Continuous use of tiny hard contact lenses for aphakia (200 cases), *Ann Ophthalmol* 5:1003, 1973.

66. Garcia GE: Continuous wear of gas permeable lenses in aphakia, *Cont and IOL Med J* 2:29, 1976.

67. Benjamin WJ, Simons MH: Extended wear of oxygen permeable rigid lenses in aphakia, *Int Cont Lens Clin* 11:547, 1984.

68. Nelson LB, Ullman S: Congenital and developmental cataracts. In Duane TD, Jaeger EA (eds): *Clinical Ophthalmology*, Philadelphia, 1988, JP Lippincott.

69. Pike MG, Jan JE, Wong PKH: Neurological and developmental findings in children with cataracts, *Am J Dis Child* 143:706, 1989.

70. Cutler SI, Nelson LB, Calhoun JH: Extended wear contact lenses in pediatric aphakia, *J Pediatr Ophthalmol Strabismus* 22:86, 1985.

71. Matsumoto E, Murphree AL: The use of silicone elastomer lenses in aphakic pediatric patients, *Int Eyecare* 2:214, 1986.

72. Neumann D, Weissman BA, Isenberg SJ, Rosebaum AL, Bateman JB: The effectiveness of daily wear contact lenses for the correction of infantile aphakia, *Arch Ophthalmol* 111:727, 1992.

73. Garcia-Kramer MY, Weissman BA: Use of tinted hydrogel contact lenses to reduce glare caused by iris abnormalities, *Int Cont Lens Clin* 19:264, 1992.

74. Crook T: Corneal infiltrates with red eye related to duration of extended wear, *J Am Optom Assoc* 56:698, 1985.

75. Herman JP: Clinical management of GPC I, *Cont Lens Spec* 2:24, 1987.

76. Zantos SG, Holden BA: Ocular changes associated with continuous wear of contact lenses, *Aust J Optom* 61:418, 1978.

77. Holden BA, Sweeny DF, Vannas A, Nilsson KT, Efron N: Effects of long-term extended contact lens wear on the human cornea, *Inv Ophthalmol Vis Sci* 26:1489, 1985.

78. Millidot M, O'Leary DJ: Effect of oxygen deprivation on corneal sensitivity, *Acta Ophthalmol* 58:434, 1980.
79. Hamano H, Hori M, Hamano T, et al: Effects of contact lens wear on the mitosis of corneal epithelium and lactate content in aqueous humor of rabbit, *Jpn J Ophthalmol* 27:451, 1983.
80. O'Leary DJ, Millidot M: Abnormal epithelial fragility in diabetes and in contact lens wear, *Acta Ophthalmol* 59:827, 1981.
81. Madigan MC, Holden BA, Kwok LS: Extended wear of contact lenses can compromise corneal epithelial adhesion, *Curr Eye Res* 6:1257, 1987.
82. Zantos SG, Holden BA: Transient endothelial changes soon after wearing soft contact lenses, *Am J Optom Physiol Opt* 54:856, 1977.
83. Schoessler JP, Woloschak MJ, Mauger TF: Corneal endothelium in veteran PMMA contact lens wearers, *Int Cont Lens Clin* 8:19, 1981.
84. Duffin RM, Weissman BA, Ueda J: Complications of extended wear hard contact lenses in rabbits, *Int Cont Lens Clin* 9:101, 1982.
85. Duffin RM, Weissman BA, Glasser DB, Pettit TH: Flurbiprofen in the treatment of corneal neovascularization induced by contact lenses, *Am J Ophthalmol* 93:607, 1982.
86. Duffin RM, Weissman BA, Elander CR, Tari L: Corneal neovascularization during HEMA contact lens wear, *Int Cont Lens Clin* 7:47, 1980.
87. Sarver MD, Sarver DS, Sarver LA: Aphakic patients' response to extended wear contact lenses, *J Am Optom Assoc* 54:249, 1983.
88. Sendele DD, Kenyon KR, Mobilia EF, Rosenthal P, Steinert R, Hanninen LA: Superior limbic keratoconjunctivitis in contact lens wearers, *Ophthalmol* 90:616, 1983.
89. Begley CG, Waggoner PJ, Hafner GS, Tokarski T, Meetz RE, Wheeler WH: Effect of rigid gas permeable contact lens wetting solutions on the rabbit corneal epithelium, *Optom Vis Sci* 68:189, 1991.
90. Mondino BJ, Groden LR: Conjunctival hyperemia and corneal infiltrates with chemically disinfected soft contact lenses, *Arch Ophthalmol* 98:1767, 1980.
91. Margulies LJ, Mannis MJ: Dendritic corneal lesions associated with soft contact lens wear, *Arch Ophthalmol* 101:1551, 1983.
92. Chun MW, Weissman BA: Compliance in contact lens care, *Am J Optom Physiol Opt* 64:274, 1987.
93. Donzis PB, Mondino BJ, Weissman BA, Bruckner DA: Microbial contamination of contact lens care systems, *Am J Ophthalmol* 104:325, 1987.
94. Weissman BA, Mondino BJ: Ulcerative bacterial keratitis. In Silbert JA (ed): *Anterior Segment Complications of Contact Lens Wear*, New York, 1994, Churchill-Livingstone.
95. Wilhelmus KR, Robinson NM, Font RA, Hamil MB, Jones DB: Fungal keratitis in contact lens wearers, *Am J Ophthalmol* 106:708, 1988.
96. Young RW: Solar radiation and age-related macular degeneration, *Surv Ophthalmol* 32:252, 1988.

Acknowledgment

I thank Kevin Miller, MD, of the faculty of the Jules Stein Eye Institute, UCLA School of Medicine, for his constructive comments on this text.

5

Postkeratoplasty Contact Lens Fitting

Anthony J. Phillips

Key Terms

keratoplasty	corneal topography	postfitting
contact lenses	postgraft fitting	complications
postgraft cornea		

The fitting of contact lenses to the postkeratoplasty patient represents perhaps the greatest challenge to the contact lens practitioner. Not only is he or she dealing with a physiologically compromised cornea, but also with the ever-present risk of graft rejection and potential eye or vision loss. In addition, the corneal topography rarely follows even a semblance of a regular pattern. Keratometry readings provide no more than a vague guide on the graft-host junction, peripheral (host) shape, or whether the graft stands proud or is tilted or sunken. Fitting demands a high level of practitioner skill and the ability to treat each patient as an individual case. Nevertheless, the postkeratoplasty patient, who has perhaps suffered from major vision loss beforehand, is often the most grateful of patients because of the visual help derived from contact lenses.

CLINICAL PEARL

The fitting of contact lenses to the postkeratoplasty patient represents perhaps the greatest challenge to the contact lens practicner.

History of Corneal Grafting

Much experimentation in corneal grafting took place during the 1800s, culminating in the first successful heteroplastic (nonhuman donor) lamellar graft by Von Hippel[1] in 1886. He used a clockwork trephine, and the patient (a little girl) had her vision improved from counting fingers to 6/60. The credit for the first full-thickness human graft that used alloplastic material and remained clear and transparent goes to Edward Zirm,[2] from the small Moravian town of Olmutz (now in Czechoslovakia). In this case the patient was blind following lime burns, and the donor was a boy whose eye had been removed because of an intraocular foreign body.

Since World War II ultrafine needles, operating microscopes, antibiotics, steroids, and improved methods of storing donor eyes and buttons have resulted in a steady increase in successful corneal graft procedures. With these aids, surgical experience and skill have increased so that the outcome of grafting procedures is now good to excellent. In recent years, techniques have evolved to reduce the corneal distortion or astigmatism so often experienced in the past, so that the end visual result is good to excellent in most cases.

Reasons for Corneal Grafting

Although some overlap exists, the reasons for grafting may be divided into physical and optical.

Physical

To Seal or to Restructure the Cornea (Tectonic Grafting)

Reasons include perforation caused by trauma or disease, and severe infections that cannot be controlled medically and may severely damage corneal rigidity.

Optical

To Restore Normal Curvature (and Therefore Refraction)

Reasons include anterior and posterior keratoconus, pellucid marginal degeneration, irregular scars caused by trauma, opaque scars caused by disease (e.g., herpes, chemical burns, benign mucosal pemphigoid, and severe keratitis sicca), and Terrien's marginal disease (which is partly tectonic and partly optical).

To Replace Corneal Opacities

Reasons include scars and chronic corneal edema such as advanced Fuchs' dystrophy and postsurgical bullous keratopathy.

The indications for corneal grafting in 3460 cases reviewed by the Australian Corneal Graft Registry in 1993[3] are set out in Table 5-1.

TABLE 5-1

Indications for Corneal Grafting in 3460 Cases Reviewed by the Australian Corneal Graft Registry in 1993

Disease/problem	Subtotal	Total	Percent
Keratoconus		1071	31%
Uncomplicated	1047		
With acute hydrops	24		
Bullous keratopathy		850	25%
Pseudophakic	577		
Aphakic	165		
Unspecified	108		
Failed previous graft		478	14%
Corneal scars and opacities		364	11%
Corneal dystrophy		234	7%
Fuchs' dystrophy	170		
Other	64		
Corneal ulcers		119	3%
Perforations	82		
Other	37		
Herpetic infection		104	3%
Active herpes simplex virus	97		
Herpes zoster			
ophthalmopathy	7		
Deformities and degenerations		54	1.5%
Descemetocele	24		
Other	30		
Keratitis		54	1.5%
Interstitial keratitis	30		
Corneal abscess	18		
Other	6		
Congenital disorders		12	<1%
Astigmatism		12	<1%
Miscellaneous		64	2%
Not recorded		44	1%

Surgical Procedure

It is not the purpose of this chapter to teach the contact lens practitioner how to perform corneal grafting, or even to understand all the surgical techniques involved. However, it is important that he or she understands the complications and difficulties of the procedure, because these often relate directly to the complications of lens fitting. Further, because patients will commonly wish to discuss surgical details with the referring practitioner, he or she should understand the procedures involved.

Keratoplasty can be done under local or general anesthesia. Adults are usually given local anesthesia, but children and the anxious are given general anesthesia.

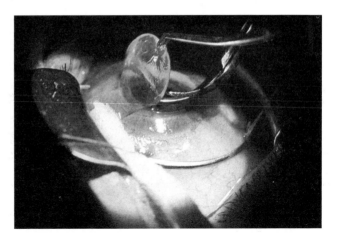

FIGURE 5-1   Removal of the opaque cornea.

Surgery is preceded by measures aimed at maintaining surgical sepsis. The eye area is cleaned and washed with surgical antiseptic, and the facial area is draped, leaving the eye exposed. In some cases a scleral ring may be sutured to the globe to give added support. This is done particularly if the patient is already aphakic, or if lens extraction is to be performed at the same time, thus reducing ocular rigidity (Figure 5-1). A trephine is selected that is large enough to remove the damaged or unwanted area.

Grafts need to be large enough for the pathology to be excised but not too large, because all things being equal, large grafts are rejected more often than smaller grafts. Small grafts may create optimal conditions for graft acceptance, but the scarred graft-host junction is more likely to produce glare and flare problems. A typical graft is 7.00 mm to 7.50 mm.

Donor corneas are obtained from the coroner after permission has been given by the relevant relative or official. Eye bank personnel also take blood from the donor and test to ensure that he or she did not carry human immunodeficiency virus (HIV) or hepatitis B virus. The excised eye is examined to ensure that the cornea is normal. The cornea, separated from the globe's posterior segment, is usually stored in tissue culture medium.

The donor button is cut from a whole eye or, more typically, from a donor cornea with scleral rim. The latter is placed front down on a nylon or Teflon block. The trephine used is typically 0.5 mm larger than the trephine used to create the graft bed. Thus a 7.5 mm trephine may be used to cut the button for a 7.0 mm graft bed. Cutting from the rear corneal surface has the effect of slightly reducing the button size, but a slightly oversized button is essential to aid graft margin sealing. It is thought that the larger graft contributes to the final myopic refraction of a higher proportion of patients having grafts for keratoconus.

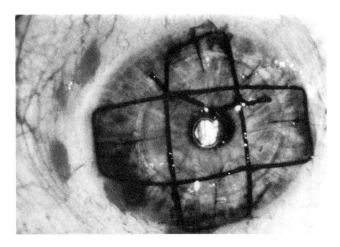

FIGURE 5-2 The four cardial sutures are shown in the 6, 12, 3, and 9 o'clock positions. The temporary fixation sutures lie over the whole corneal surface.

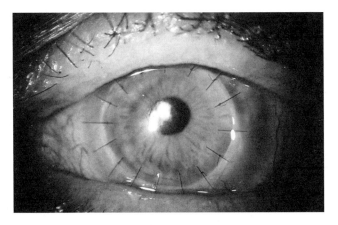

FIGURE 5-3 An example of interrupted sutures in a corneal graft.

The surgeon now returns to the recipient cornea and trephines all the way through or, more typically, approximately 85% of the way through the corneal thickness. Final cutting is done with a sharp blade or scissors to remove the unwanted cornea. By angling the scissors, a small rear surface ledge may be created to support the donor button.

The donor cornea is placed in the recipient bed and four cardinal sutures are placed in the 12, 6, 3, and 9 o'clock positions (Figure 5-2). Fine 10-0 nylon is used. After the donor cornea is secured, further suturing is done. These may include an additional 8 to 12 interrupted sutures (Figure 5-3), a continuous suture (Figure 5-4), or a combination of both single and interrupted sutures. Although each surgeon will have his or her preferred suturing method, interrupted sutures

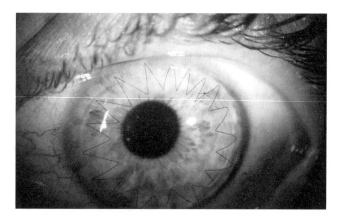

FIGURE 5-4 An example of a single or continuous suture around a penetrating graft.

are generally used if the wound may be expected to heal unevenly, such as in a vascularized cornea or where vessels may rapidly enter along an individual suture line. In this case the single suture can easily be removed. It is claimed that a combination of continuous and interrupted sutures enables control of astigmatism because a single or double interrupted suture can be removed should a high astigmatic error appear, leaving the graft supported by the continuous suture. The cardinal sutures may or may not be removed after the placement of the continuous suture.

If the surgery has been uneventful, the patient is discharged the same day, or after 2 or 3 days hospital bed rest and observation.

Postoperative Management

Grafts done for dystrophic conditions such as keratoconus seldom reject, but grafts done for postinflammatory disease reject more often. Allograft rejection is the most common cause of corneal graft failure.

The risk of graft rejection is greatest in the first year and falls steadily thereafter, although the patient should be warned that graft rejection always remains a possibility. To minimize graft rejection, patients are given topical steroid drops for at least 3 to 6 months, and often longer. Corneal healing is slow and sutures are usually left in place for at least 12 months. Even after a year, wound healing may be incomplete. As a general rule, sutures are left in place beyond 12 months if the keratometer readings are reasonably regular and without excessive (<6.0 D) astigmatism, and if minimal or no host vascularization occurs to the graft margin. Conversely, if marked graft distortion, excessive astigmatism, or neovascularization to the graft margin or into the graft is present, the sutures are generally removed as soon as wound healing looks adequate, but seldom earlier than 12 months. Loose or broken sutures are removed early. If there are no optical, discomfort, or rejection episodes, appointment intervals are gradually widened until the sutures are removed, typically at 12 to 18 months. Thereafter, patients are reviewed annually by the surgeon.

Rejection Episodes

All eye care professionals should be aware of the signs and symptoms of graft rejection. Rejection episodes are most likely in the first year after surgery and become less frequent thereafter. If caught early, steroid treatment is often all that is necessary, and the graft can be saved in the majority of cases. If left for several days or longer, the risk of total graft failure becomes very high. The warning sign of rejection is inflammation with a subsequent drop in vision.

All inflammatory episodes in corneal transplant patients must be taken seriously, because inflammation often precedes rejection. Because an inflammatory response and new vessel growth can be a complication of contact lens wear, practitioners must be careful to identify and rectify these processes, because they almost always precede rejection. It must be impressed on patients that any ocular inflammation necessitates immediate lens removal and indicates the need to see their practitioner as soon as possible. The effect of inflammation on the outcome of grafting is shown dramatically in Figures 5-5 and 5-6.[4]

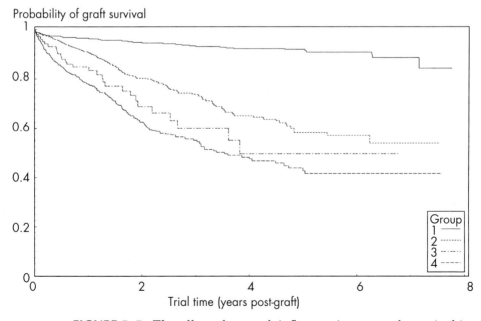

Probability of graft survival

Trial time (years post-graft)

FIGURE 5-5 The effect of pregraft inflammation on graft survival in 4349 cases. *Group 1,* host never inflamed; *Group 2,* host not inflamed at grafting but inflamed in the past; *Group 3,* inflamed at grafting but not in the past; *Group 4,* inflamed at graft and also in the past. (Source: Australian Corneal Graft Register, 1994).

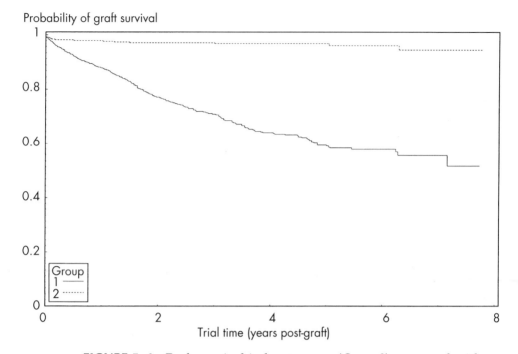

Probability of graft survival

Trial time (years post-graft)

FIGURE 5-6 Graft survival in keratoconus (*Group 2*) compared with corneal grafts done for all other reasons (*Group 1*) (N = 4499 cases). The high survival rate of noninflamed keratoconic eyes is striking.

Raised intraocular pressure is another cause of graft failure. It may arise because of preexisting glaucoma, anterior segment inflammation, or the use of corticosteroid eye drops. A close watch should therefore be kept on intraocular pressure.

Finally, it should be borne in mind that the risk of allograft rejection increases with the number of grafts performed on the same eye (Figure 5-7).[5]

Numbers of Procedures Performed

Woodward[6] notes that approximately 1400 transplants are performed each year in the United Kingdom. Casey and Mayer[7] give an annual figure of 12,500 in the United States in 1984; Coster and Williams[8] estimate this number currently at 30,000, and give figures of 1500 for Australia, Germany, and Japan. The number of procedures is steadily increasing over the world, but in many countries religious beliefs inhibit or prohibit donation of eyes.

The reported percentage of postkeratoplasty patients requiring contact lens correction varies considerably in the literature. Ruben and Colebrook[9] give a figure of 65% for a series of 100 grafts for

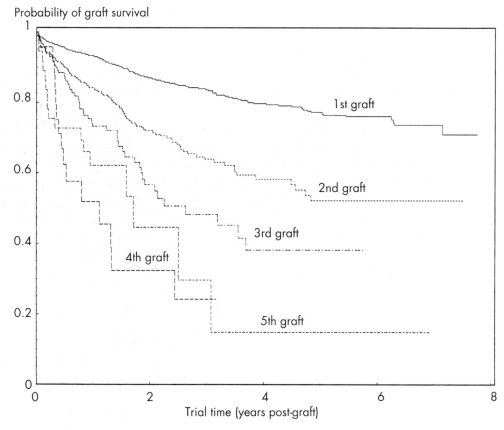

Probability of graft survival

Trial time (years post-graft)

FIGURE 5-7 Graft survival of second grafts is poorer than of first grafts; third and subsequent grafts are poorer again. The probability of graft survival at 2 years between first and multiple grafts is 30%. (Source: The Australian Corneal Graft Registry Annual Report, 1994).

keratoconus because of the resulting high astigmatism. Conversely, Brightwell and Laux[10] give a figure of 16% for 199 consecutive cases; Cohen and Adams[11] give a figure of 10%. As surgical techniques improve, the number of patients requiring a contact lens is steadily falling (Table 5-2). Because this is counteracted by the increasing number of keratoplasty procedures being performed, the true figure has not fallen so dramatically.

Postgraft Cornea

Keratoplasty Thickness

Immediately after transplantation, the donor button may be extremely edematous, with the thickness gradually returning to normal levels over days or weeks. In the first year postgraft (while steroids are still

TABLE 5-2

Methods of Postgraft Visual Correction*

Method of Correction	Total	Failed	Surviving
Glasses only	1176	37	1139
Contact lens only	211	1	210
IOL only			
PC IOL	471	125	346
Sutured PC IOL	87	19	68
AC IOL	232	81	151
Iris IOL	36	24	12
Unknown IOL	54	12	42
Glasses and contact lens	52	1	51
Glasses and IOL			
PC IOL	603	29	574
Sutured PC IOL	134	5	129
AC IOL	178	25	153
Iris IOL	40	13	27
Unknown IOL	19		19
Contact lens and IOL			
PC IOL	10	2	8
Sutured PC IOL	2		2
AC IOL	8	2	6
Iris IOL			
Unknown IOL	1		1
Glasses and contact lens and IOL			
PC IOL	6		6
Sutured PC IOL	1	1	
AC IOL	2		2
Iris IOL			
Unknown IOL	1		1
No correction/not recorded	1175	263	912
TOTALS	4499	640	3859

*Just under 50% of all patients have spectacles, 42% have an IOL in place, and nearly 7% have contact lenses. More than one refracting device is in use by 24% of recipients (Source: Australian Corneal Graft Registry Annual Report, 1994).

being used and the sutures are in situ), the grafted cornea may be thinner than normal.[12] However, if corneal thickness is measured when treatment has ceased and the sutures have been removed, the vast majority of grafts are thicker than normal. Ruben et al,[13] in a study of 51 successfully grafted eyes, showed an average graft thickness of 0.60 mm and only 15% of grafts within normal limits of thickness. There was no correlation between the age of the graft and thickness, but correlation was found between visual acuity and graft thickness, visual acuity falling significantly when the cornea was thicker than 0.62 mm. The implication of these findings is that even with successful clear grafts, the majority are slightly edematous even before the application of a contact lens.

The graft tissue's essential contribution is the endothelium. Although the donor's epithelium and stromal cells may be replaced by host cells, the grafted endothelium persists and is the metabolic powerhouse of the cornea. The graft's survival depends on the endothelium's survival, and the general state of the endothelium should be carefully checked before lens fitting commences.

Graft Endothelial Morphology

Brown and Bron[14] showed that in many successful clear grafts individual endothelial cells are much enlarged. It is thought that most endothelial cell damage occurs at the time of surgery, with more cells lost from the peripheral graft and recipient cornea nearer the junction than from the central graft. The central graft cell population reduces as cells migrate toward the peripheral zone, enlarging in the process. This slow process of cellular reorientation lasts approximately 3 years. Bourne[11] and Ruben et al,[12] studying the same group of patients, showed a mean cell count of $1226.02 + 393.84/mm^2$ cells for their graft count, compared to $3233.62 + 328.38/mm^2$ for a matched control group.

Although corneal thickness near normal limits may be maintained with endothelial cell counts less than one third of normal, clinical experience indicates that a cornea with a low endothelial cell density is more vulnerable to extraneous conditions that might induce corneal edema. Thus care must be taken in the choice of lens material and in lens fitting so that the contact lens' occlusive effect does not trigger an edematous response with which the cornea cannot cope. Fortunately, Speaker et al[15] have shown that well-fitting RGP lenses of high Dk/t have little or no effect on graft endothelial cell survival in the first few years after surgery.

Graft Sensitivity

Ruben and Colebrook[9] measured the corneal sensitivity of 50 successfully grafted eyes using the Cochet and Bonnet anesthesiometer. Their findings are shown in Table 5-3.

In the normal cornea, central sensitivity is considerably greater than that of the corneal periphery, but on a typical grafted eye the reverse applies. Other findings by these researchers showed that 14.6% of the grafted eyes showed no measurable central sensation and

---

Table 5-3

Results of Ruben and Colebrook on Corneal Sensitivity of Grafted Eyes

Corneal Position	Maximum Mean Length of Monofilament Just Felt
Graft center	1.80 cm
Host (peripheral) cornea*	2.66 cm

*A normal center reading is 4.0 cm.

that no instances of normal corneal sensation were found until at least 3 years after surgery.

The last finding is significant because most patients fitted with contact lenses tend to be fitted fairly soon after sutures are removed (that is, anything from 6 to 18 months after keratoplasty). This means that the majority of patients are fitted when central corneal sensation is significantly reduced, if not absent. Furthermore, Millodot[16] has shown that contact lens wear depresses corneal sensation even further.

Although corneal sensation and the normal warning signals of abnormal changes are reduced, lid sensation is not. Thus the postkeratoplasty patient is as sensitive, if not more so, than the nongrafted patient. Indeed, psychological problems are often encountered that may appear to exacerbate symptoms of sensitivity, because often the postgraft patient had hoped to avoid the need for a contact lens. Nevertheless, patients do not experience the normal discomfort produced by a corneal abrasion or edema. The symptoms denoting corneal edema about which grafted patients sometimes complain are nearly always visual.

Graft Topography

When grafts are examined by photokeratoscopy, it is rare to find a regular surface contour. The effect of differing curves of host and graft, suturing, operative technique, oversizing of graft, and the healing process all combine to produce a complex surface. Fitting is not easy with any type of lens. Compromise fittings and the ability to design a lens for each patient are essential. Nevertheless, graft shapes can be divided into several general headings, and an understanding of these is useful.

CLINICAL PEARL

The effect of differing curves of host and graft, suturing, operative technique, oversizing of graft, and the healing process all combine to produce a complex surface.

Nipplelike Protrusion

Most grafts are steeper than the host cornea and protrude slightly in a nipplelike manner (Figures 5-8 and 5-9). This protuberance has been attributed to the second anchor zone of collagen produced by scarring at the donor-host junction, coupled with the lower rigidity of the graft itself, or to its increased thickness and higher water content, or both. As stated earlier, most grafts are effectively oversized by 0.2 mm to 0.3 mm to provide a better donor-host junction seal. This oversizing also exacerbates graft protuberance.

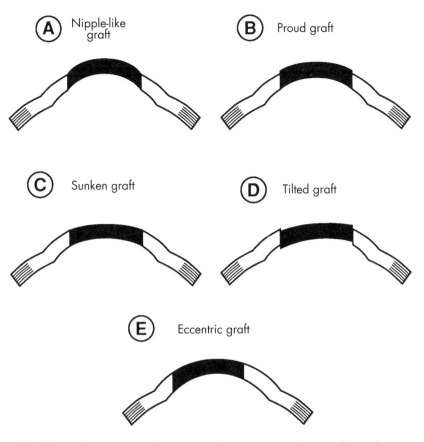

FIGURE 5-8 A to E, Diagrammatic representations of postkeratoplasty corneal topography as it relates to contact lens fitting.

Proud Grafts

Grafts that stand slightly proud of host cornea cause particular problems to the contact lens practitioner (see Figures 5-8 and 5-10). Rigid lenses, which are frequently necessary to provide adequate vision, often will fall off the graft when displaced by lid action. Large or reverse geometry lenses are often essential in such cases.

Proud grafts are commonly produced for the same reasons as nipplelike protrusions, but are possibly more common in keratoconic grafts, where the host margin may be thinner than normal or where the surgeon has entered the graft and host with the needle at unequal levels at opposing points. A shelved cut in the host cornea also can produce a proud graft. It should be emphasized that a proud graft is rarely visible by slit-lamp biomicroscopy, but is readily visible by examination of the contact lens fluorescein pattern.

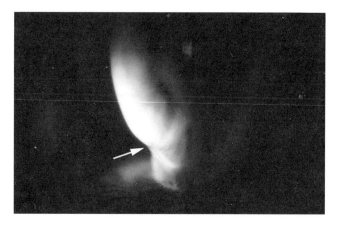

FIGURE 5-9 A nipplelike graft showing the steepening in corneal curvature at the host-graft junction *(arrow)*.

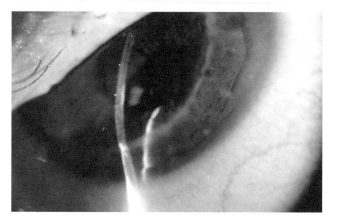

FIGURE 5-10 A proud graft showing a raised step at the host-graft interface.

Sunken Grafts

If the graft and recipient bed are of the same or very similar size, a sunken graft may result (see Figure 5-8, C). Although poor unaided vision may ensue, these cases are generally easier to fit than proud grafts because a rigid lens can be used to vault the sunken area. Fenestrating the lens is occasionally necessary if retrolens bubbles occur in more markedly sunken grafts.

Tilted Grafts

A graft may register only low or moderate astigmatism when measured with the keratometer, yet when a corneal contact lens is fitted it will not center and shows excessive stand-off in one area. This usually is caused by the graft being tilted in relation to the host cornea (see Figure 5-8). This may be produced by variations in the host or graft margin thickness, or in the suture depth between graft and host around the graft.

If a contact lens is large enough to bridge the graft, there will be a localized tear guttering effect. Tilted grafts present a severe problem to the contact lens practitioner and it is difficult to avoid persistent bubbles over a recessed area. However, a stationary bubble can soon induce neovascularization and must be avoided.

Eccentric Grafts

When grafting a keratoconic eye, most surgeons center the graft on the thinnest part of the cornea, which is commonly not on the visual axis (see Figure 5-8). In the case of corneal scarring the graft is usually centered on what was the most densely scarred area. The implication of this is that a lens designed to center on the graft may well be off-the eye's visual axis.

Graft Toricity

One of the major factors affecting vision in the postkeratoplasty patient is moderate, high, or irregular astigmatism. Astigmatic errors as high as 10.0 D to 15.0 D are not uncommon, with 6.0 D considered typical. Astigmatism can arise for a variety of reasons, most of which require a high level of skill (and a certain amount of luck!) on the part of the surgeon if they are to be avoided. For example, incorrect placement of the first four cardinal sutures will result in unequal distribution of graft tissue; incorrect radiality of the sutures will induce a torque effect in the graft, unequal suture tension can produce high corneal cylinders, preexisting astigmatism in the host or cornea can be a problem, and a preexisting corneal scar can produce tension within the stroma so that a circularly trephined cut produces an oval hole.

Surgical Reduction of Postkeratoplasty Astigmatism

In cases of nonvascularized grafts exhibiting high astigmatism in which a spectacle correction may not be tolerated or contact lens fitting may be difficult, surgical intervention may improve corneal topography.

Using local anesthesia and photokeratoscopy for guidance, the surgeon may make two "relaxing incisions" some 90% through the graft margin in an arc around the steepest graft meridian. Further suturing of the incisions is not necessary, although three "compression sutures" are sometimes inserted on each side along the flatter meridian to steepen it during the healing process.

In severe astigmatism, a small wedge of tissue may be removed from each of the graft margin's two flatter corneal meridians to

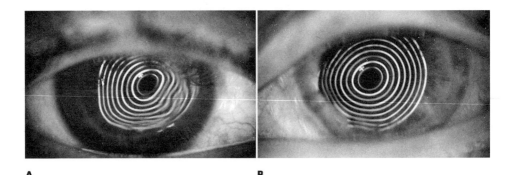

A   **B**

FIGURE 5-11 The effect of relaxing incisions in reducing 10.0 D corneal astigmatism is shown by comparing the photokeratographs in **A** and **B**. Peripheral distortion is still clearly visible, but reasonable spherical central images can be seen. In other cases little or no change occurs after relaxing incisions.

provide a "wedge resection" and thereby steepen the graft along this meridian.

Such operative procedures provide no guarantee of success, but usually reduce the higher levels of astigmatism (Figure 5-11).

Fitting Procedures

No set pattern or lens type is ideal in the postkeratoplasty situation, although rigid gas-permeable lenses undoubtedly predominate. Each patient must be assessed in a holistic fashion and warned from the outset that some experimentation may be necessary to achieve the desired result. Factors to be borne in mind will be discussed in the following sections.

CLINICAL PEARL

No set pattern or lens type is ideal in the postkeratoplasty situation, although rigid gas-permeable lenses undoubtedly predominate

Physiological Limitations of the Grafted Cornea

Factors such as vascularization in or near the graft, significant endothelial cell loss, or whether it is a first, second, or third graft should always be remembered.

Psychological Attitude of the Patient

Many patients may have previously worn contact lenses and are often precipitated into grafting because of problems in lens fitting, such as in advanced keratoconus. Their last experience of contact lens wear thus may have been neither successful nor happy. Further, although surgeons invariably warn prospective keratoplasty patients that the possibility exists that contact lenses may be essential to restore normal vision after grafting, there is no doubt that a proportion of patients undergo grafting in the hope of avoiding contact lens wear. Knowing that lens fitting also is unlikely to be easy or straightforward means that a positive attitude toward success is always necessary, even though the complexity of fitting should be discussed where appropriate.

Whether Fitting Is to Be Done With Sutures Present or Removed

Lens fitting is normally contraindicated if sutures are still present, and definitely for 4 to 5 months after surgery (longer in the case of older patients, where healing is slower). However, in cases such as a monocular grafted patient with high postsurgical graft distortion or toricity, fitting over or between the sutures may be essential. In such cases a thin soft lens, a small rigid gas-permeable (RGP) lens fitted within the sutures, a large lens with a bearing surface beyond the sutures, or even a piggyback combination may be necessary.

It is essential when fitting over sutures that the eye not be hyperemic, that the graft be clear, that good vision be achievable with an acceptable overrefraction, and that the patient be able to return for frequent follow-up visits.

Time After Suture Removal

The majority of grafts become more regular with time. It is, therefore, usual for the eye to require refitting at least once in the first 3 years.

Lens fitting is not normally commenced until at least 2 to 4 weeks after suture removal. Fitting can be commenced earlier in younger patients, who generally heal quicker.

Fitting Set Availability

The almost infinite variety of graft, host, and junction shape permutations means that the design of appropriate fitting sets becomes impossible. Although conventional lenses often work successfully, most lenses, particularly in RGP designs, are custom made for the individual patient. Because two or three lenses for each eye are often necessary to achieve a correct (and usually compromise) fit, a fitting set of unwanted trial lenses will usually be accumulated over a period of time. Postgraft fitting is therefore best left to the practitioner who wishes to specialize in this area.

Prefitting Examination

A normal contact lens prefitting examination should be carried out with particular attention to the following:
1. Full refraction and note of the best acuity obtained. Acuity at low contrast sensitivity also is ideal where possible. The improvement

over these readings will determine the value of contact lens fitting or whether spectacles alone may be applicable (unless contact lenses are requested for cosmetic purposes or are necessary for correction of marked anisometropia).

2. Careful note should be made of any sutures present; whether these are completely buried (i.e., epithelialized) or not; if any likelihood exists of suture protrusion that could damage a soft lens or cause marked discomfort; the presence and extent of neovascularization; the topography of the graft margin and the symmetry of the graft position; the graft's state and clarity; and the state and quality of the graft endothelium. A photographic record in addition to the visual examination is always ideal.

3. Keratometry readings should be taken and the degree of distortion noted. If available, photokeratoscopy also should be performed, because this sometimes gives clues as to the topography of the graft-host interface zone. Although keratometry readings may serve as a rough guide, they give no significant indication as to the back optic zone radius (BOZR) of the optimum lens fit.

Rigid Gas-Permeable Lenses

The majority of postkeratoplasty patients are fitted with RGP lenses. The reason is usually the poorer acuity obtained with soft lenses over the irregular and often highly astigmatic graft-host cornea. Physiological factors such as significant graft endothelial loss or neovascularization to the graft margin or just into the graft also may indicate RGP fitting. High Dk gas-permeable material is used to minimize any anoxic stress, and such lenses are worn almost invariably, on a daily-wear basis only. As with soft lenses, several approaches to fitting are possible and more than one may have to be adopted for a successful conclusion. The prefitting examination will give the first indication of the technique likely to prove optimal.

Conventional Lenses

In regular and near regular grafts (particularly in grafts of long standing) where the corneal curvature begins to approach normal, a conventional fitting technique may be employed. Often a toric back surface is necessary. For the practitioner new to postkeratoplasty fitting, this simple approach should always be made first, because not only is it sometimes applicable (often unexpectedly so), but also a regular curved lens will usually give a topographical picture of the whole corneal surface (Figure 5-12). From this, a more logical decision as to the next step can be made.

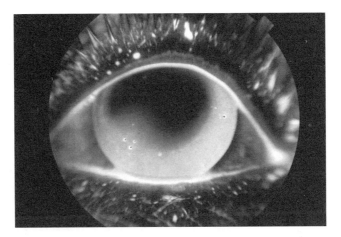

FIGURE 5-12 A conventional, large tricurve lens fitted onto a proud graft showing graft alignment and excessive peripheral clearance.

Fitting Over Sutures

Fitting over sutures is best avoided because of potential fitting and physiological complications. At best, the lens is likely to be of temporary value only, because the fitting will undoubtedly change after the sutures are removed. Nevertheless, for those cases in which fitting over sutures becomes necessary, several approaches may be adopted:

1. Because of the raised area of graft-host interface and sutures, a thin soft lens may be tried first; this may drape over the raised doughnut area without producing bubbles in the central graft area. However, poor acuity caused by lens distortion often necessitates the use of an RGP lens.

2. Fitting a large lens over the suture zone to bear on the peripheral host cornea usually provides a stable lens and good acuity. The fitting of these larger lenses is described later in the chapter. The main disadvantages are the occlusive effects of these larger diameter lenses and the introduction of bubbles under the central graft area as the lens is lifted up by the often raised interface-suture area. Fenestrating this area may help, but is not often successful.

3. Thin small RGP lenses fitted within the suture line may be helpful. Such lenses are usually 6.00 mm to 6.50 mm total diameter and of single or bicurve construction. Their main disadvantages are handling problems, mediocre comfort in many cases, and a tendency to displace easily.

4. Other lens designs or combinations such as silicone lenses or piggyback designs, may be experimented with if all else fails. In

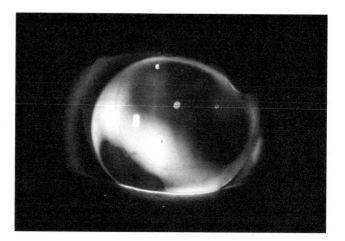

FIGURE 5-13 An example of a sunken graft along the 135-degree axis. An acceptable area of alignment has been maintained over the rest of the graft and host with fenestrations positioned so that at least one is over the proud area to aid tear interchange.

the case of piggyback designs the adverse effect of reduced oxygen permeability on the relatively new graft should not be forgotten.

Sunken Grafts

The fitting procedure here is in many respects similar to postradial keratotomy (post-RK) fitting, except that the peripheral cornea retains its normal shape. A large (9.50 mm to 10.50 mm total diameter) conventional fitting can be employed, with care being taken to provide sufficient peripheral bearing in much the same way as keratoconus or post-RK fitting techniques. Fenestrations may be employed where there is marked pooling to prevent tear liquid stagnation (Figure 5-13).

Proud, Tilted, or Displaced Grafts

The combination of slightly thick grafts in thin (usually keratoconic) hosts means that grafts commonly stand proud of the surrounding host area. A 2 μm to 3 μm step is sufficient to allow displacement of a conventionally fitted lens, which then sits grossly displaced from the visual axis. In such cases a large RGP lens or one of the alternative lens forms becomes necessary (Figures 5-14 to 5-17).

In the days of PMMA lenses, large lens designs almost invariably produced graft edema even if fenestrations were incorporated to improve tear exchange. The advent of high Dk RGP materials has allowed much greater use of these designs.

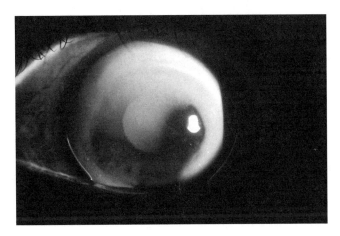

FIGURE 5-14 An inferiorly proud or tilted graft fitted with a 10.50 mm total diameter lens to provide inferior graft matching and superior host alignment.

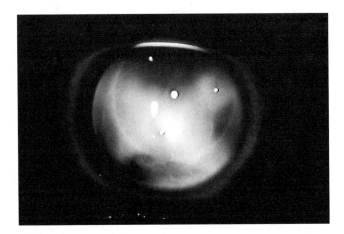

FIGURE 5-15 An example of a markedly proud graft in the horizontal meridian. In this instance a large (12.00 mm) diameter corneal lens has been fitted with a narrow peripheral band of alignment. The lens vaults over the proud areas to make gentle contact and has two fenestrations to aid tear interchange.

These larger lenses vary between 10.0 mm and 12.0 mm and are commonly of simple tricurve and quadricurve design. Because the intention is to span the graft and the irregular host-donor junction, it is essential that the BOZD be larger than the graft itself. Currently, the majority of grafts have diameters between 7.0 mm and 8.0 mm. Thus the BOZDs of lenses prescribed vary between 8.0 mm and 10.0 mm.

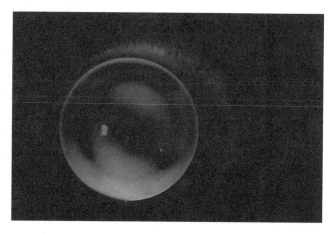

FIGURE 5-16 A toroidal graft showing a nearly spherical host.

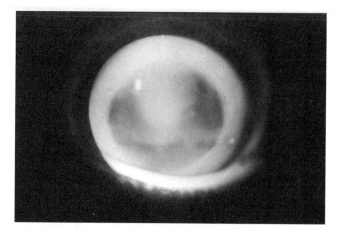

FIGURE 5-17 A proud graft has been fitted with a large (12.00 mm) total diameter lens to give graft and outer peripheral alignment. Four fenestrations (three visible) have been placed in the clearance band between graft and aligning periphery to aid tear interchange.

With a BOZD of 8.00 mm or 9.00 mm in a tricurve lens of 10.0 mm total diameter, the second curve usually needs to be approximately 1.00 mm flatter (e.g., 8.10:8.00/9.10:9.50/11.00:10.00); with larger lenses, the flattening needs to be greater (e.g., 8.20:9.50/10.00:11.00/12.25:11.50 or 8.20:10.00/11.00:11.50/13.50:12.00).

It is almost impossible to design fitting sets for postkeratoplasty fitting. Most practitioners build one up from unsuccessful lenses. Nevertheless, the use of trial lenses is absolutely essential in these cases.

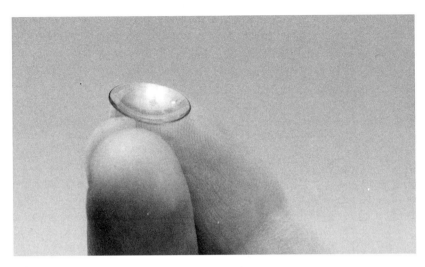

FIGURE 5-18 Balancing a large diameter corneal lens on one finger can be difficult for both practitioner and patient. Insertion devices may be used or, as shown here, the lens may be balanced on the tips of two fingers.

Problems with larger lens designs will be discussed in the following sections.

Patient Handling

Although a large lens may be balanced on a fingertip as with smaller conventional designs, it often is helpful to use a suction holder or suspend a lens between two adjacent fingertips (Figure 5-18). Lens removal can be effected by the normal stare-pull-blink technique in some cases, but is best done by either using a suction holder or by the two finger stretch technique (Figure 5-19). Here the upper lid is pressed against the globe with the index finger of one hand while the lower lid is pressed against the globe by the index finger of the other hand. The lids are then stretched toward the ear in an arc just above and below the lens. If gentle pressure is kept against the globe, the lids should be forced behind the lens and the lens ejected as the arc is completed.

Lack of Lens Movement

This is one of the major problems with large lens designs, particularly as the total diameter approaches the corneal diameter. Even with high Dk materials, corneal staining will result from an immobile lens. The use of fenestrations, a smaller total diameter, flatter peripheral curves, lubricant drops, and even a regular manipulation of the patient's lid to enforce lens movement may be necessary. If these actions fail, alternative lens forms should be used.

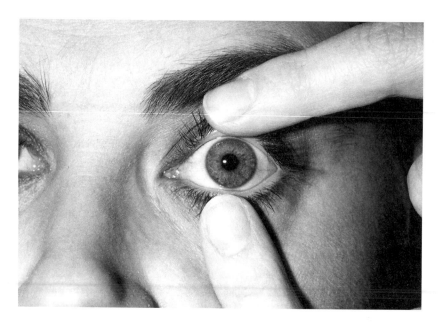

FIGURE 5-19 To remove large diameter corneal lenses, the stare-blink technique often does not work because the lid aperture cannot be opened wide enough. In these cases either a suction holder or the two finger technique shown here should be used. This technique involves pressing the lid margins gently against the eye with the fingers arcing outward above and below the lens. By pressing the lids against the eye and stretching them tight, the lens should be ejected.

Bubbles Around the Graft Margin

These may arise around the graft margin of proud grafts or in the gutter zones of tilted grafts. Fenestrations are the answer in most cases. Persistent bubbles may cause slight patient discomfort and also may provide a stimulus for neovascularization by producing localized xerosis. In extreme cases scleral lenses or piggyback designs may be necessary.

A further advance in lens design for the proud graft is the steep secondary curve lens. The development of advanced computer numeric controlled (CNC) lathes has enabled laboratories to produce lenses with peripheral curves steeper than the BOZR. Significant improvements in lens stability, comfort, and retrolens tear flow have occurred since these designs became available. Two of the most useful are the OK84 and OK85 designs by Contex. These lenses have secondary curves 4 D and 5 D (0.8 mm and 1.0 mm) steeper respectively than the BOZR and a third, flatter, aspheric periphery. The lens is fitted to align with the graft and with the third (BPR_2) curve aligning the host. The author uses a trial set of the OK85 design with BOZRs ranging from 6.5 mm to 8.00 mm and total diameters of

11.50 mm. Two grafted corneas fitted with OK85A lenses are shown in Plate 19. Sometimes up to a 9.0 D steeper secondary curve is necessary.

Use of Corneal Mapping Devices in Fitting RGP Lenses

Corneal mapping devices such as the EyeSys or TMS-2 have proven helpful in fitting complex corneas such as postgraft corneas. Plate 20 illustrates such a case.

Plate 20 shows the cornea's tangential plot using EyeSys. The graft is markedly proud with a steep, clearly demarcated border and flat host. The graft shows with-the-rule astigmatism and is tilted on the temporal edge. The keratometric data is shown in Plate 33. An OK84 or OK85 (Contex) design was selected to provide the best fit. The best aligning lens is that averaged over the whole graft surface (i.e., typically 7.0 mm or 7.50 mm diameter). The average curvature on the numeric plot for 7.0 mm (the edge of the graft) is 7.76 mm. Frequently, an OK84 or OK85 lens of this BOZR shows excellent alignment. In this instance, a simulated lens fitting using fluorescein may allow refinements to the fit before trying a lens on the eye (Plate 20).

It was expected that the lens would center over the proud temporal edge; the "Pan R/L" control was therefore set to position the lens with a 0.5 mm temporal lens decentration. The "Tilt" was set on Auto. The OK85 has an 8.00 mm BOZD and a 1.0 mm steeper secondary curve. Unfortunately, the present EyeSys program does not allow wide enough secondary and tertiary curve widths to simulate the typical 11.50 mm total diameter lens. Nevertheless, it was obvious that the theoretical 7.76 BOZR lens would be too flat and that a 7.40 BOZR would provide a better compromise fit. The effect of lid pressure and the corneal molding thereby produced showed a much greater area of apparent alignment with the same trial lens on the eye.

Soft (Hydrogel) Lenses

Soft (hydrogel) lenses are fitted relatively infrequently in postkeratoplasty cases for four reasons:

1. The relatively high resultant astigmatic error after grafting in the majority of cases is undesirable. Stock toroidal lenses are rarely suitable.
2. The general irregularity of the new corneal surface, with differing curves of graft and host combined with the possibility of a raised host-graft junction, or a proud, tilted, or sunken graft makes fitting difficult. These factors often combine to produce distortion in any design of soft lens used.
3. The greater occlusive effect of soft lenses compared with smaller gas-permeable hard lenses, especially over the peripheral host area, can lead to neovascularization in the host and eventually into the graft, and also to graft edema, especially if significant endothelial loss has occurred. Both situations may trigger graft

rejection, and regular aftercare and patient instruction are of paramount importance.

4. The possibility exists of wide fluctuations in vision, because the cornea changes shape if soft lenses are fitted early after grafting or suture removal.

It should be emphasized that once having been fitted with a hydrogel lens, postgraft patients often do not take kindly to being fitted with RGP lenses that initially produce a greater foreign body sensation. For example, grafts that shift in the host bed after initial lens wear and that later necessitate an RGP lens to correct the induced astigmatism, often produce discomfort out of proportion to that normally experienced. Thus soft lenses should only be contemplated when physiological or visual symptoms or sensitivity strongly indicate their use.

Three approaches may be used in the fitting of hydrogel lenses:

1. In cases of hypersensitivity to rigid lenses, or perhaps where a tint or prosthetic design is needed, conventional fitting can be tried. Trial lenses equating to the best sphere should be tried. The thickness of the trial lens should equal that of the final lens, and an overrefraction should be performed after 1 hour of lens wear. The residual cylinder and visual acuity achieved can be assessed and the decision made whether or not to proceed with a hydrogel lens. A custom-made toric lens is almost always necessary. Zonal (reversed prism) thinning designs rather than prism ballast designs should be used; these are preferable physiologically because of the reduced lens thickness. A medium water content lens also is preferable for physiological reasons, but should always be worn on a daily-wear basis to avoid graft hypoxia that could trigger a rejection response. With present generation materials, extended wear should only be contemplated in the cases of thin, plano therapeutic lenses or aphakic keratoplasty patients with cystoid macular edema.

2. In a case in which the fitting of a soft lens is essential or preferable but where the corneal surface is irregular, a slightly thicker than normal hydrogel lens may help improve otherwise poor acuity. Conventional hydroxyethyl methylacrylate (HEMA) or medium water content designs may be used, but with thicknesses that are double or triple the conventional ultrathin thicknesses for the same power. Such lenses must be used with great care, regular monitoring, and lens wear usually restricted to part-day wear only. Hydrogel lenses are more successfully employed in aphakic keratoplasty cases in which the anterior segment physiological demand is reduced and the natural increase in lens thickness at these powers often masks any corneal irregularity.

3. Piggyback lens designs also are useful. These are discussed in the next section.

Extended-wear soft lenses are best avoided for all postkeratoplasty patients because of the dangers of neovascularization.[17] The only exception may be for aphakic keratoplasty patients who have had cystoid macular edema. In such cases resulting poor vision prevents daily lens insertion, and extended wear may be the only practical solution. Nevertheless, extended wear should still be approached with great care and regular monitoring. The use of high Dk rigid gas-permeable lenses is preferable where possible, because the risk of neovascularization is reduced.

Combination or Piggyback Lenses

In cases of gross irregularity or irregular astigmatism, or in cases in which excessive lid margin sensitivity is present, the combined use of soft and rigid lenses may be considered.[18-21] The soft lens provides a more regular and comfortable base over which a high Dk RGP lens is fitted to provide good acuity. By smoothing out surface irregularities such as proud or tilted grafts, RGP fitting is simplified and problems of grossly displaced lenses are thereby avoided (Figure 5-20).

In keratoconus a similar problem exists, and here a high negative-powered soft lens is commonly used as a carrier to more nearly produce a normal surface curvature on which to fit the RGP lens. In the postkeratoplasty situation, a much wider variety of corneal shapes may be present. Where possible, a low positive-powered, lenticulated, mid water content hydrogel lens is used as the combination base. Use of a mid water content soft lens and high Dk RGP material is essential to avoid graft edema and neovascularization. The soft lens is fitted in the normal way, with excessive movement avoided by increasing the

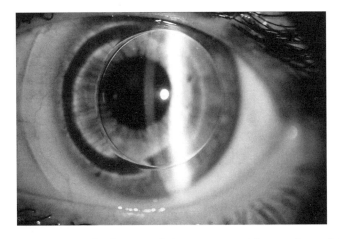

FIGURE 5-20 An RGP lens sunk into a recess of a carrier soft lens.

total diameter. After the soft lens has settled, front surface keratometer readings are taken to provide information for the RGP fitting. Use of a lenticulated positive-powered lens aids centration of the RGP lens that also may be fitted slightly on the tight side to avoid excess movement or RGP displacement. Because of the underlying soft lens material, a good tear pump action is obtained and discomfort is rare. Simple bicurve or tricurve designs are normally adequate.

Supplementary spectacles may be sensible if the total power of rigid and soft combination results in too great an overall thickness to significantly reduce the combined transmissibility. The main problems with this system are the risk of graft edema and neovascularization, and the cost and nuisance factor of two lenses in one eye.

Scleral Lenses

Although fitted by only a few practitioners (usually in hospital settings), scleral lenses are still of value in postkeratoplasty because they have the following advantages:
1. They are easily handled, even by persons with severe arthritis.
2. They are almost impossible to lose.
3. Centration is good whatever the degree of corneal irregularity.
4. Good levels of vision are the norm.
5. They have a long lens life.
6. They are simple to maintain and carry little risk of giant papillary conjunctivitis (GPC).

The corneal molding or impression technique is the preferred method of fitting. The back optic zone curvature often is chosen by using trial and error to find the best diamond grinding tool that takes up the irregular back surface of the impression shell. The full technique is described in detail by Pullum.[22]

The main disadvantages of scleral lenses in the postkeratoplasty situation are:
1. Corneal edema, often with the absence of any discomfort.
2. Neovascularization. Regular aftercare is of paramount importance.
3. The time and difficulty in fitting.

Silicone Lenses

Silicone rubber has been investigated as a material for contact lenses for nearly three decades. Its main attractions are its high oxygen permeability and, in the postkeratoplasty situation, its greater rigidity providing a higher acuity.

The advantages of silicone rubber lenses follow:
1. Very high oxygen permeability
2. Better or more stable acuity than soft lenses
3. Greater comfort than RGP lenses in hypersensitive cases
4. Good centration even in cases of gross corneal irregularity or decentered grafts

5. Less variation in comfort or fit under differing environmental conditions, or in cases of accompanying dry eye

The disadvantages of silicone rubber lenses include the following:

1. They are difficult to fit, requiring as much or greater precision than rigid lenses, and a longer time to settle.
2. A negative pressure effect may occur, particularly if the lenses are not fitted correctly, so that some lenses have a tendency to stick to the cornea.
3. The lenses have a short lifespan because of breakdown in the surface coating and build-up of deposits.
4. Difficulties with surface wetting are possible.
5. The lenses have a restricted range of parameters.

SoftPerm Lens (Formerly Known as the Saturn Lens)

In cases of markedly decentered grafts, highly irregular corneal topography, other grossly decentered lens fits, or highly sensitive eyes, the SoftPerm lens may be indicated.[23,24]

The SoftPerm lens consists of a rigid gas-permeable center of 8.0 mm diameter made of a silicone-acrylate tertiary butylstyrene copolymer surrounded by a soft 25% water content HEMA hydrophilic skirt of 14.3 mm diameter. The BOZR of the central zone varies from 6.70 mm to 8.10 mm. The hydrophilic skirt enables good lens centration and significantly improves comfort. Such a lens design offers the best long-term solution for these difficult cases. The main problems are cost, limited parameters, lack of adequate lens movement on postkeratoplasty eyes, mediocre physiological properties, and physical strength at the material interface.

Other Lens Designs

Materials have been developed over the last ten years that cannot be defined strictly as RGP or as soft lenses. One such material is the UltraCon* lens, which may best be described as a firm yet flexible gas-permeable (FGP) lens.

The UltraCon lens has been developed from a polymer originally developed to oxygenate blood during heart/lung surgery. Its manufacturers claim the material is more durable than a typical hydrogel lens and can be manufactured in varying degrees of flexibility from rigid to soft. Manufacture is by molding with six BOZRs, a total diameter of 13.00 mm, and BVP range of −8.00 D to +6.00 D in 0.25 D steps. The Dk varies from 80 to more than 150 depending upon the degree of relative flexibility, which (with a nominal center thickness in minus powers of 0.10 mm) gives an excellent Dk/t.[25,26]

Although the lens is flexible (resembling a hydrogel lens), no water is necessary and in this respect the lens is more typical of a conventional

---

*Ultra Vision, Inc.

RGP lens. A high refractive index (approximately 1.50) and low specific gravity (approximately 1.01, increasing as the flexibility decreases) with excellent surface wettability are claimed.

The relative rigidity (compared to a hydrogel lens) means that the lens corrects a wide range of corneal astigmatic errors. Lens handling is similar to a soft lens, except that a suction holder may be used if necessary.

The EpiCon* lens uses the same material as the UltraCon lens, but is made in slightly more rigid form (Dk approximately 50 to 100). The total diameter is 13.50 mm, resembling a small soft lens. The back surface typically has a 7.20 to 8.00 spherical BOZR, an intermediate aspheric zone, and a spherical periphery zone. Eight BOZRs are available, each with three edge lifts, so that sagittal depths can be varied to control lens fit. The lens may be fenestrated (0.2 mm to 0.5 mm) to assist in the removal of retrolens debris and to create a tear pump action between the lens and the eye. The EpiCon lens finds particular use in pathological eye situations such as keratoconus, high corneal cylinders, Terrien's marginal disease, and pellucid marginal degeneration.

Advantages

1. Excellent oxygen permeability
2. More comfortable than other RGP lenses in the adaptive phase
3. Less easily lost than the conventional RGP designs
4. Masks corneal cylinders better than standard hydrogel lenses (up to 300 D claimed)
5. Good wetting properties and deposit resistance
6. Not susceptible to dehydration on the eye, unlike normal hydrogel lenses
7. Wide range of pathological eye applications
8. Conventional fluorescein can be used to check lens fit

Disadvantages

1. The material is new at the time of writing and possible long-term problems are unknown.
2. There is a limited range of parameters.
3. Astigmatism other than corneal astigmatism cannot be corrected.
4. The lens design does not encompass sophisticated designs (e.g., bifocals).
5. Patients with narrow vertical interpalpebral apertures will still find smaller conventional RGP designs easier to handle.
6. A suction holder is normally needed to remove the lens.

---

*Specialty Contact Lens Ltd.

Therapeutic Uses of Contact Lenses in the Postkeratoplasty Situation

1. Woodward[27] and Manabe et al[28] have commented that the postgraft use of contact lenses helps mold the corneal surface, thereby reducing corneal irregularity.
2. Casey and Mayer[7] note that some surgeons have used a soft lens to maintain the anterior chamber while they sutured through a cut-out in the lens periphery.
3. Therapeutic soft lenses can protect uncomfortable sutures if the surgeon is unwilling to risk resuturing or removing the sutures.
4. In those patients whose epithelial healing is impaired (e.g., from ocular surface abnormalities such as Stevens-Johnson syndrome, chemical burns, or herpetic keratitis), it is important to provide good epithelial cover as soon as possible. Although a young donor with intact epithelium is the essential factor, a thin bandage lens can help prevent epithelial trauma caused by the lids during blinking.
5. Usually a small leak can be sealed with a bandage lens without surgical intervention. The edges will be held in place and edema may seal the leak under the lens. The lens can usually be dispensed with after a few days if necessary.
6. Ingrown lashes can have a devastating effect on graft epithelium and should be dealt with before surgery. However, if they develop or are missed clinically, a bandage soft lens will serve as protection.

It cannot be overstressed that great caution should be used in the application of bandage lenses while the cornea is immunosuppressed and completely denervated.[29]

Complications of Fitting

Lens wear may have to be discontinued for the reasons discussed in the following sections.

Graft rejection

Lens wear should be discontinued immediately if graft rejection is detected or even suspected. Cautious readaptation may commence after the condition is controlled, but if rejection episodes recur, lens wear may have to be ceased permanently or some significant improvement made in lens design or material to achieve greater oxygen permeability. Graft rejection is more likely if previous grafts have been performed on the same eye.

Inadequate Vision

Even with RGP lenses, there may be inadequate gain over conventional spectacle correction to justify contact lens wear. In other cases an astigmatic lens may locate obliquely or at right angles to the central astigmatism, as indicated by keratometry leaving high residual astigmatic error that may be almost impossible for laboratory fabrication.

Graft Neovascularization or Edema

Neovascularization into the graft or graft edema may necessitate discontinuation of lens wear. However, improvements in lens design or material may be tried first before rejecting lens wear altogether. Consultation with the graft surgeon also is a sensible precaution.

Lens Intolerance

As with all contact lens wearers, the occasional hypersensitive patient may not be able to successfully tolerate a lens. With the choice of lenses now available these patients are decreasing in number, but in some cases a gain in lens comfort may have to be set against a decrease in vision by using alternative methods of correction.

Corneal Ulcers

Although they are rare, researchers have reported corneal ulcers in contact lens wearers.[19,20] The effect on a corneal graft patient can be disastrous and reinforces the need for careful patient instruction and monitoring.

Fees and Charges

It is essential from the outset that patients be warned that postkeratoplasty contact lens fitting may be simple and straightforward, or extremely complicated and time consuming. Further, patients should be told that the determination of the ultimate lens may be quickly achieved or may only result from the trial of several lens designs and types. Considerable skill and experience are required on the part of the fitter.

The significantly longer time and greater number of lenses used in the majority of cases, combined with more expensive high Dk material, inevitably result in higher fees and charges. Patients should be counseled about this before fitting commences.

Conclusion

The improvement in surgical techniques has reduced the number of postkeratoplasty patients requiring contact lenses for visual rehabilitation. This reduction has been partially offset by the increasing numbers of grafts being performed. Further, those patients requiring contact lenses usually need complex of fittings and are in the greatest need of contact lens correction. The services of a good contact lens practitioner are indispensable to the corneal graft surgeon.

CLINICAL PEARL

The services of a good contact lens practioner are indispensable to the corneal graft surgeon.

Postkeratoplasty fitting presents perhaps the greatest challenge to the contact lens practitioner. Every facet of fitting skill, lens design, visual optics, knowledge of corneal physiology, and results of corneal surgery and its complications is called on. However, for patients who have undergone the major surgical and psychological trauma of a corneal graft, the end visual result is extremely worthwhile. Postgraft patients maintain a strong loyalty to their surgeons and contact lens fitters.

References

1. Von Hippel A, Albrecht V: *Graefes Arch Ophthalmol* 34:108-112, 1888.
2. Zirm E, Albrecht V: *Graefes Arch Ophthalmol* 64:580-584, 1906.
3. Williams KA, Muehlberg SM, Wing SJ, Coster DJ: The Australian corneal graft registry, 1990-1992 report, *Aust N Z J Ophthalmol* 21 (suppl): 1-48, 1993.
4. Williams KA, Muehlberg SM, Lewis RF, Coster DJ: How successful is corneal transplantation? A report from the Australian corneal graft register, *Eye* 9:217-219, 1995.
5. Williams KA, Muehlberg SM, Lewis RF, Coster DJ: Graft survival after corneal transplantation. On behalf of all contributors to the Australian Corneal Graft Registry (ACGR), *Transplant Proc* 27:2141-2142, 1995.
6. Woodward EG: Post-keratoplasty. In Phillips AJ, Stone J (eds): *Contact lenses,* ed 3, London, 1989, Butterworths, 764-772.
7. Casey TA, Mayer DJ: Contact lenses post keratoplasty. In *Corneal grafting—principles and practice,* ed 1, Philadelphia, 1984, WB Saunders, 281-288.
8. Coster DJ, and Williams KA: Donor cornea procurement; some special problems in Asia, *Asia Pac J Ophthalmol* 4, 2, 7-12, 1992.
9. Ruben M, Colebrook E: Keratoconus, keratoplasty curvatures and lens wear, *Br J Ophthalmol* 63:268-273, 1979.
10. Brightbill FS, Laux DJ: Contact lens fitting. In *Corneal surgery—theory, technique, and tissue,* St Louis, 1986, Mosby, 344-351.
11. Cohen EJ, Adams CP: Postkeratoplasty fitting for visual rehabilitation. In Dabezies, OH (ed): *The CLAO guide to basic science and clinical practice,* vol. 2, Orlando, 1984, Grune and Stratton, 52.1-52.7.
12. Bourne WM: Morphologic and functional evaluation of the transplanted human cornea, *Trans Am Ophthalmol Soc* 81:403-450, 1983.
13. Ruben M, Colebrook E, Guillon M: Keratoconus, keratoplasty, thickness, and endothelial morphology, *Br J Ophthalmol* 63:790-793, 1979.

14. Brown NAP, Bron AJ: Endothelium of the corneal graft, *Trans Ophthalmol Soc UK* 94:863-870, 1974.
15. Speaker MG, Cohen EJ, Edelhauser HF, Clemens, CS, Arentsen JJ, Laibson PR, Raskin EM: Effects of gas permeable contact lenses on the endothelium of corneal transplants, *Arch Ophthalmol* 1703-1706, 1991.
16. Millodot M: Corneal sensitivity and contact lenses, *Optician* 162:23-24, 1971.
17. Cunha MC, Thomasson TS, Cohen EJ, et al: Complications associated with soft contact lens use, *CLAO* 13(2):107-111, 1987.
18. Baldone JA: The fitting of hard contact lenses onto soft contact lenses in certain diseased conditions, *Cont Lens Med Bull* 6:15-17, 1973.
19. Baldone JA: Piggyback fitting. In: Dabezies O H (ed): *Contact Lenses—The CLAO guide to basic science and clinical practice*, vol. 2, Orlando, 1984, Grune and Stratton.
20. Caroline PJ, Doughman DJ: A new piggyback lens design for correction of irregular astigmatism—a preliminary report, *Cont IOL Med J* 1979;5:40-42.
21. Soper JW, Paton D: A piggy-back contact lens system for corneal transplants and other cases with high astigmatism, *Cont IOL Med J* 6:132-134, 1980.
22. Pullum K: Eye impressions, production and fitting of scleral lenses and patient management. In Philips AJ, Stone J (eds): *Contact Lenses*, ed 3, London, 1989, Butterworths 645-702.
23. Astin C: The use of Saturn II lenses following penetrating keratoplasty, *Trans Br Cont Lens Conf* 2-5, 1985.
24. Zilliox J: Fitting the Saturn II, *Cont Lens Forum* 54-57, December 1985.
25. Hammock G: A new approach to correcting astigmatism, *Spectrum* 42-44, October 1993.
26. Sturm B: Development of the UltraCon and EpiCon, *Optical Prism* 25-28, January 1994.
27. Woodward EG: Contact lens fitting after keratoplasty, *J Br Cont Lens Assoc* 4(2):42-49, 1982.
28. Manabe R, Matsuda M, Suda T: Photokeratoscopy in fitting contact lens after penetrating keratoplasty, *Br J Ophthalmol* 70:55-59, 1986.
29. Saini JS, Rao GN, Aquavella JV: Post-keratoplasty corneal ulcers and bandage lenses, *Acta Ophthalmol* 66:99-103, 1988.

Bibliography

Aquavella JV: Factors affecting vision following keratoplasty noted, *Ophthalmol Times* 29, Jan. 1989.
Aquavella JV, Shaw EL: Hydrophilic bandages in penetrating keratoplasty, *Ann Ophthalmol* 8:1207-1219, 1976.
Binder PS, Zavala EY, Deg JK, Baumgartner SD: Hydrophilic lenses for refractive keratoplasty: the use of factory lathed materials, *CLAO* 10:105-111, 1984.
Cavanagh D, Leveille A: Extended-wear contact lenses in patients with corneal grafts and aphakia, *Am Acad Ophthalmol* 89:643-650, 1982.
Constad W: Fitting post-op keratoplasty patients with RGP CL's, *Cont Lens Forum* 11:40-48, 1988.
Contact lenses assist visual recovery after keratoplasty, *Ophthalmol Times*, April 1986.
Cowden J: Continuous wear aphakic soft contact lenses following keratoplasty, *Ann Ophthalmol* 579-582, May 1980.
Dangel ME, Kracher GP, Stark WJ: Aphakic extended wear contact lenses after penetrating keratoplasty, *Am J Ophthalmol* 95:156-160, 1983.
Daniel R: Fitting contact lenses after keratoplasty, *Br J Ophthalmol* 60:263-265, 1976.
Daniel R: Post keratoplasty fitting of contact lenses, *Cont Lens J* 5:6-8, 1977.
Ekuful SM: Using soft toric lens to correct high astigmatism after penetrating keratoplasty, *Cont Lens J* 16(4):76-77, 1988.

Genvert G, Cohen E, Arentsen J, Laibson P: Fitting gas permeable contact lenses after penetrating keratoplasty, *Am J Ophthalmol* 99:511-514, 1985.

Hom MM: The challenge of fitting corneal transplants, *Cont Lens Forum* 60-64, Nov. 1985.

Jensen AD, Maumenee AE: Refractive errors following keratoplasty, *Trans Am Ophthalmol Soc 1974* 72:123-131, 1979.

Lemp MA: The effect of extended wear aphakic hydrophilic contact lenses after penetrating keratoplasty, *Am J Ophthalmol* 90:331-335, 1980.

Mannis M, Matsumoto E: Extended wear aphakic soft contact lenses after penetrating keratoplasty, *Arch Ophthalmol* 101:1225-1229, 1983.

Mannis MJ, Zadnik K, Deutch D: Rigid contact lens wear in the corneal transplant patient, *CLAO* 12(1):39-42, 1986.

Moore JW: Contact lens fitting after penetrating keratoplasty, *Cont Lens Forum* 38-42, Aug. 1986.

Paglen PG, Fine M, Abbot RC, Webster RG: The prognosis for keratoplasty in keratoconus, *Ophthalmol* 89:651-654, 1982.

Rao GN, John T, Ishida N, Aquavella JV: Return of corneal sensitivity in grafts following penetrating keratoplasty, *Ophthalmol* 92:1408-1411, 1985.

Samples J, Binder P: Visual acuity, refractive error, and astigmatism following corneal transplantation for pseudophakic bullous keratopathy, *Ophthalmol* 92:11, 1985.

Smiddy WE, Hamburg TR, Kracher GP, Stark WJ: Keratoconus. Contact lens or keratoplasty?, *Ophthalmol* 95:487-492, 1988.

Soper JW: Fitting corneal transplants with corneal contact lenses, *Int Cont Lens J* 3:31-35, 1976.

Soper JW, Jarrett A: Results of a systematic approach to fitting keratoconus and corneal transplants, *Con Cont Lens J* 9:12-22-22, 1975.

Troutman RC: Astigmatism considerations in corneal grafts, *Ophthalmic Surg* 10:21-26, 1979.

Zadnik K: Post-surgical contact lens alternatives, *Int Cont Lens Clin* 15:211-220, 1988.

Acknowledgements

The author wishes to thank the following for their help in the preparation of this chapter: Professor Douglas Coster, Head of the Ophthalmology Department, Flinders Medical Center, Adelaide; Wendy Laffer, for constructive comments on the manuscript; Glenn Boucher of the Illustration and Media Department, Flinders Medical Center; and Eva Lefty, for typing and manuscript layout.

6

Contact Lenses and Refractive Surgery

Joseph P. Shovlin, Michael D. DePaolis,
James V. Aquavella

Key Terms

refractive surgery	wound healing	neovascularization
informed consent	contact lens base	residual refractive
radial keratotomy	curve	error
photorefractive	contact lens	
keratectomy	complications	

For almost 200 years, ophthalmic surgeons have tried to correct refractive error with means other than spectacles and contact lenses. Initial attempts were rudimentary and fraught with disaster. Even today, refractive surgery remains the most controversial ophthalmic surgical procedure performed.[1]

However, several procedures have evolved into legitimate options for a select group of patients. This chapter will briefly review the procedures in use today, and the role that contact lenses play for patients undergoing them.

The postrefractive surgery cornea has a more aberrant optical performance than its preoperative counterpart.[2] In fact, all of the refractive procedures attempted to date share the optical complications of glare, photophobia, undercorrection and overcorrection, induction of regular and irregular astigmatism, loss of best visual acuity, regression of effect, and monocular diplopia. Eyeglasses, contact lenses, or repeat surgery can help correct many of these complications.

Lans was the first to perform incisional corneal surgery in 1898. Lans' work went largely undetected until 1939, when Sato began his work, leading the way for expansion into surface area techniques. The procedure was first performed on diseased (keratoconus) rather than myopic eyes. By inducing surgical hydrops through endothelial side incisions, significant flattening of the eccentric cone occurred after several weeks of pressure patching.

Sato's procedure for keratoconus ultimately led to the correction of astigmatism and eventually to the correction of myopia. His early attempts to correct myopia required as many as 32 incisions on the anterior and posterior surfaces to achieve a greater effect (Plate 21). In spite of these multiple incisions and a constant 6 mm optic zone, he achieved an average correction of just 3 diopters (D).[1]

In general, posterior corneal incisions produce little change because the index of refraction between the cornea and the aqueous is so similar. Furthermore, as many as 80% of the corneas followed in Sato's case series at the University of Juntendo have decompensated.[1] This is particularly significant because it occurred in a population virtually immune to Fuch's dystrophy or other endothelial dystrophies. Nearly all the cases decompensated at about 40 years of age, irrespective of the patient's age at the time of surgery.[1,3]

Credit for the later interest in and success of radial keratotomy (RK) goes to S. N. Fyodorov, a prominent Russian ophthalmologist. His reports in the late 1970s aroused much interest in the United States. Fyodorov claims that in a group of patients with between 1 D and 3 D of myopia, 100% had visual acuities of 20/50 or better without correction following his technique; 85% achieved 20/25 or better.[1,3]

Bores and Gould of the United States began offering the first instructional course for RK in 1980 after making several trips to Russia in the late 1970s.[1] A prospective evaluation of radial keratotomy (PERK) study funded by the National Institutes of Health enrolled 450 patients from eight university centers across the United States.[4-6] The study, including results and possible complications, will be evaluated later in this chapter.

RK and other surface area techniques (e.g., relaxing incisions, wedge resections, and other augmentation methods for postpenetrating keratoplasty patients) have evolved greatly since Sato's initial work. Some of the dramatic changes include more well-defined algorithms and nomograms, a reduction in the number of incisions, and changes in direction of cut (downhill followed by uphill), blade material and design (duotrack), pachymetry techniques (interferometry), and topographic assessment.[1,3] One of the most significant trends is toward shorter and fewer incisions (Figure 6-1).

A   **B**

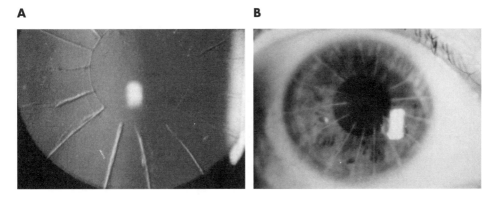

FIGURE 6-1 **A,** Retroillumination shows a 16-incision radial keratotomy performed around 1980. **B,** Diffuse illumination highlights an old 16-incision radial keratotomy.

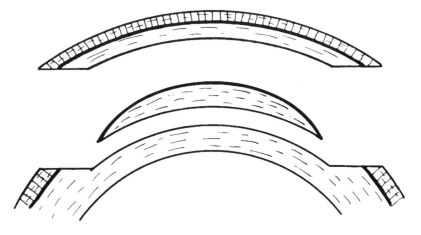

FIGURE 6-2 This schematic depicts the stromal section required in keratophakia, a thickness volume technique.

Thickness volume techniques, including keratomileusis, keratophakia (stromal inlays), epikeratoplasty, and automated lamellar keratoplasty (ALK) are procedures that have evolved from corneal surface modifications pioneered by Barraquer and Ruiz. He recognized that to achieve permanent change in corneal curvature it was necessary to add or excise corneal tissue.

Barraquer and Ruiz are credited with virtually all the initial work in the fields of keratomileusis and keratophakia (Figure 6-2), both lathing procedures. As a result of these complex and difficult procedures, other areas of refractive surgery have developed. Herbert

Kaufman is given credit for a so-called "reversible" procedure (epikeratoplasty), whereby a lamellar onlay is placed on the recipient bed to correct high refractive errors such as keratoconus (Plate 22). Epikeratoplasty is rarely performed today. Because of the complex and unreliable nature of keratomileusis and keratoplasty, ALK has gained popularity recently. In this procedure a microkeratome is passed through the cornea at the midstromal level. The corneal cap is then flipped over and a second microkeratome pass is made to remove stromal tissue and effect a power change. In a variation of ALK known as laser assisted in-situ keratomileusis (LASIK), an excimer laser is used to contour the exposed stromal bed, in a procedure referred to as "flap and zap."

These advances have decreased the number and seriousness of complications, and to a certain extent improved predictability. Unfortunately, there are now nearly as many viable techniques as surgeons performing them.[1] Even successful procedures can leave the patient with uncorrected residual refractive error and occasional irregular astigmatism. These misadventures require spectacles, contact lenses and, occasionally, excimer laser photorefractive keratectomy (PRK) for correction.

Refractive surgery, in all its various forms, is still in its early stages. In the future, surgical correction of refractive error for most may be an acceptable alternative to the use of optical devices.[1] With the advent of PRK, LASIK, and ALK, early techniques are becoming obsolete and refractive surgery is being recognized as a mainstream option. Major changes are expected in the not-so-distant future, including new laser procedures. Core studies with sighted eyes for several excimer and non-excimer lasers are already underway.

Trends

Although the number of exotic procedures such as keratomileusis and epikeratoplasty has declined in recent years, the number of RK procedures has steadily increased. Optimistic 10-year PERK study results and pending FDA appoval of the excimer laser have piqued an interest in refractive surgery. Most major cities have at least a few ophthalmic surgeons who regularly perform refractive surgery.

Although they may not necessarily possess a "guinea pig" mentality, patients who pursue refractive surgery are often adventure seekers[7] who are fearful of myopia and have an abhorrence of spectacles. Erickson has identified potential refractive surgery candidates as being auditorily based, associative, and tolerant of a certain amount of risk.[8]

In the last 5 to 7 years, refractive surgical procedures have undergone dramatic modification and improvement. As the procedures evolved, the complications associated with them decreased. Still, the most frequently encountered complication following all refractive surgical procedures is overcorrection and undercorrection.[1,3,5,6] In RK, for example, undercorrection occurs with much greater frequency than overcorrection, especially in eyes with more than 6 D of myopia. As surgeons have become more experienced with RK, the percentage of patients with less than 4 D of myopia that are corrected close to emmetropia appears to be increasing.[1,9] This can be attributed to a surgical titration in which the RK surgeon employs a conservative primary technique followed by enhancement as needed. Unfortunately, RK is hampered by a propensity towards hyperopic shift. In this scenario the patient manifests an excellent initial result, but becomes progressively hyperopic over time.

Whereas undercorrection seems to be more common with epikeratoplasty, the reported cases of undercorrection and overcorrection seem about equal with keratophakia and with myopic and hyperopic keratomileusis.[3,10,11]

Perhaps the most consistent refractive surgery technique is PRK. Although still in its infancy, PRK is as accurate and predictable as the most refined RK procedures.[12] In fact, the potential for further refractive error refinement through repeated ablations is evident.[13]

Although ALK and LASIK show great promise, particularly for greater degrees of myopia, there is a relative dearth of long-term, large series data.

Medico-Legal Aspects

The litigious society in which we live requires that ophthalmic practitioners consider the risks of recommending or performing refractive surgery. Some will be called on to rectify a residuum of a refractive surgery misadventure. Because these patients are often disgruntled, practitioners must proceed with caution. It must be remembered that elective procedures carry a greater legal hazard than required procedures or those without better alternatives.[1] The procedure's hazards vary compared with the alternatives—spectacles, contact lenses, and intraocular lenses.

Some complications of refractive surgery (e.g., glare, uncertainty of final outcome, and fluctuation in acuity)[1] are not serious. These complications may be tolerable, but more serious complications such as cataract formation, keratitis, endophthalmitis, and vascularization may threaten vision or globe integrity (Figure 6-3). These catastrophies, including the possibility of endophthalmitis following perforation with RK, present a serious threat of litigation.[1] Generally, patients who are intolerant of optical devices are more likely to sue than the more phlegmatic types.[1] Many candidates for refractive surgery also have unrealistically high expectations.

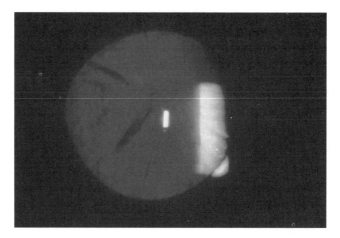

FIGURE 6-3 Cataract formation has occurred in this patient following frank perforation. Retroillumination shows spokelike opacity of the crystalline lens.

The need for truly informed consent is greatly increased with elective procedures.[14] In cases such as refractive keratoplasty fully informed consent is essential. Printed forms to educate the patient are acceptable, but do not substitute for the personal exchange between practitioner and patient.[1,14]

In procedures such as refractive keratoplasty the practitioner recommending the procedure may have the patient write out what he or she understands of the procedure and its risks on his or her patient chart after a personal interview.[1] After a thorough discussion of the procedure, patients can take a self-assessment test to better gauge their understanding of risks and benefits. If any misunderstandings persist, they can be rewritten by the patient on his or her chart. A patient who is properly and fully informed rarely sues.

Other factors vital in reducing the likelihood of litigation are full and open communication, a properly trained and pleasant staff, good records, and early consultation when warranted.[1] It is essential to inform each patient of the worst case scenario.

Good records are essential because they reflect what transpires and are not subject to the fallacies of memory.[1] A record should never be altered in such a way that the scratched-out material cannot be read, nor should anything be added after a patient has filed a claim.[1] Such changes can easily be detected[1,6] and can make the case indefensible.[1,14]

In light of the medico-legal implications it is prudent to consider a presurgical contact lens fitting for demonstration purposes. By employing disposable hydrogel lenses, the clinician can demonstrate the effects of residual astigmatism, myopia, and monovision to prospective refractive surgery patients. Through this method there can be no misunderstanding regarding visual outcomes.

In fitting contact lenses following refractive surgery, the fitter may be vulnerable to litigation even if he or she did not perform the procedure. Several late-presenting complications may occur and (at least in theory) may be precipitated or aggravated by contact lens wear. Adequate insurance coverage is essential for the practitioner who recommends or performs refractive surgery or who is called upon to follow or rehabilitate the cornea afterward. The amount of coverage should be no less than $1 million per event.[1]

Refractive surgery may be relatively new, but the safest ethical and legal approach to it is an old one—always do what is in the patient's best interest without regard to finances, personal aggrandizement, or benefit to the practitioner. The potential risks and benefits must always be considered.

Although the scientific basis for refractive surgery's efficacy may rest upon the patient achieving good visual acuity (20/40 or better), in the final analysis success depends on a satisfied patient.[1] Much of the groundwork is laid before the procedure is even performed. Overpromotion of refractive surgery as a means of eliminating optical devices can only increase the chances of having a dissatisfied patient whose expectations are not and could not have been met.[1]

CLINICAL PEARL

Overpromotion of refractive surgery as a means of eliminating optical devices can only increase the chances of having a dissatisfied patient whose expectations are not and could not have been met.

Surgical Options

To better understand the corneal changes (topographical hysteresis) that take place during refractive surgery, a review of past and present procedures will be provided.[15]

Thickness Volume Techniques

Keratomileusis

Keratomileusis is a refractive lamellar autokeratoplasty. It changes spherical refractive defects by altering the radius of the curvature of the cornea's anterior face. In the operating room, a complex lathe precisely grinds the patient's cornea, modifying its thickness by removing a lamellar disc of corneal collagen. After the patient's disc is removed, it is submitted to the action of cryopreserving solutions, or "frozen." The lamella's posterior face is ground according to measurements obtained preoperatively, including keratometry, refractive error, and intraocular pressure. The lathed disc is then returned to the stromal bed and sutured into place. Keratomileusis may be used to correct myopia or hyperopia. In myopia, the lathe disc becomes the negative lens, whereas in hyperopia, the disc becomes the positive lens. Keratomileusis is generally reserved for those with high refractive error and anisometropia.

As in most forms of refractive surgery, certain contraindications exist. For keratomileusis these contraindications include keratitis sicca, ocular surface disease, keratoconus and distorted corneas, thin corneas (<0.45 mm), excessively flat (>8.50 mm) or steep (<7.30 mm) corneas, glaucoma, and dense amblyopia.

Although amblyopia is always a diagnosis by exclusion and a relative contraindication to all refractive surgery, there actually may be some benefit for these individuals. By placing the refractive correction in the corneal plane much as with contact lenses, retinal imagery may be improved.

No donor tissue is used in keratomileusis.

Keratophakia

An intralamellar donor lenticule of plus power is inserted into host stromal pocket. The stromal lenticule is lathed preoperatively, so no complex intraoperative manipulations are necessary. A microkeratome and suction ring are used to cut off the host cornea's cap. The lenticule is inserted, after which a running 10-0 nylon closure is done in the standard fashion. Keratophakia is generally limited to high hyperopia, primarily aphakia. Contraindications to keratophakia are the same as those for keratomileusis.

Donor tissue is necessary for keratophakia.

Epikeratoplasty

In this procedure superficial epithelium is meticulously removed and a small defect (keratectomy) is made in Bowman's membrane and the superficial stroma. A preground lyophilized or frozen lenticule is placed on the corneal surface and sutured into the host stroma. The lyophilization or freezing kills the lenticule's keratocytes; ultimately, the patient's cells invade this donor cornea and epithelium grows over it. This in effect provides a living contact lens that can be removed if complications develop.

Although the indications for epikeratoplasty are similar to keratomileusis and keratoplasty, epikeratoplasty is rarely performed. Its primary indications are for high hyperopia and anisometropia, especially monocular aphakia in children. A secondary indication is for keratoconus.

Contraindications for epikeratoplasty are similar to those for keratomileusis. In addition, the procedure should be avoided in keratoconus if apical scarring exists. Potential complications of epikeratoplasty include persistent epithelial defects, interfacial epithelial ingrowth, interfacial neovascularization, and a decentered button with induced astigmatism.

Because of the potential complications associated with epikeratoplasty, this technique has become less popular in recent years. Its viability in the surgical correction of keratoconus and pediatric aphakia remain.

Donor tissue is required for epikeratoplasty.

Automated Lamellar Keratoplasty (ALK)

In recent years the previously discussed thickness volume techniques have given way to ALK. Although similar in principle, ALK is less technically complex and requires no donor tissue. In ALK, the surgeon stabilizes the globe with a microkeratome-based suction ring. An initial microkeratome pass is made to resect a plano layer of corneal tissue at the anterior one-third stromal level. The surgeon is careful not to complete the keratome pass, but instead leaves a small hinge of attached cornea so the corneal cap can be flipped over. In this fashion the surgeon has an exposed stromal bed for subsequent resections. The microkeratome is then reset and an additional "power" resection is made to change the refractive error. Some surgeons use excimer laser ablation to make the necessary refractive error change, in a procedure referred to as "flap and zap" or LASIK. At this point, the corneal cap is flipped back over onto the stromal bed, and the eye is pressure patched over an antibiotic application.

Indications for ALK include high myopia, hyperopia, and anisometropia. ALK is contraindicated for those with ocular surface disease, keratitis sicca, distorted corneas (as in keratoconus), glaucoma, and amblyopia.

Although considered a fairly safe and effective procedure, certain complications can ensue after ALK. In the immediate postoperative phase a chance of corneal cap displacement exists, and stromal scarring and irregular astigmatism can complicate ultimate visual outcome.

No donor tissue is required for ALK.

Intrastromal Inlays

Current research is assessing the viability of hydrogel and other synthetic materials to obviate the need for human donor tissue. Although early research with primates has been encouraging, biocompatibility with the donor tissue remains a long-term obstacle. In intrastromal inlays, a synthetic lenticule is inserted into a stromal pocket. If a material with a higher index of refraction than that of the cornea is used (i.e., polysulfone), little anterior surface change is needed (Figure 6-4). Whenever material with a similar index of refraction is used (i.e., hydrogel), a significant anterior bulge or flattening, depending on the desired correction, is needed to effect

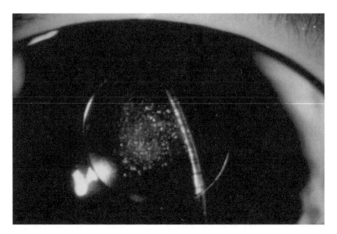

FIGURE 6-4 A polysulfone inlay used many years ago often resulted in anterior corneal opacity.

refractive change. Clinical applications for intrastromal inlay have yet to be well defined.

Donor tissue is necessary for intrastromal inlay.

Surface Area Techniques

Corneal Wedge Resection

Corneal wedge resections have gained little popularity as a means of reducing large amounts of astigmatism. They work by steepening the flat meridian and flattening the steep meridian. A crescentic lamellar incision is made for approximately 25% of the corneal graft circumference. The incision is deepened to full cornea[1] thickness and an adjacent angled incision is made. The wedge is then sutured to create a steepening effect. For every 0.1 mm of tissue removed, astigmatism is reduced approximately 1.0 D. Although sound in principle, it is extremely difficult to accurately assess tissue reduction. The potential for perforation, infection, and poor refractive results have made corneal wedge resection a rarely performed procedure today.

Corneal Relaxing Incisions

Relaxing incisions are often used to reduce high astigmatism following keratoplasty. In this procedure no lamellar wedge of tissue is removed. Full thickness incisions are made to Descemet's membrane, most often within the host-graft junction, effectively creating a new limbus and a wound gape that flattens the cornea's steeper meridian. As with wedge resection, the flatter meridian is secondarily steepened. A Ruiz procedure uses tangential incisions along the steepest meridian to flatten the cornea; a compensatory steepening occurs along the flattest meridian (Figure 6-5). Occasionally, augmentation (compressive) sutures are used in the flattest meridian, 90 D away

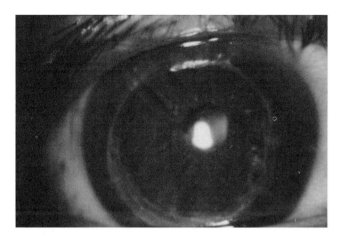

FIGURE 6-5 Ruiz incisions (tangential) are shown following a successful corneal transplant. Unfortunately, high astigmatism resulted and an attempt at flattening the steepest meridian was undertaken. This procedure is not commonly used today.

from the relaxing incisions. Relaxing incisions are usually performed under the biomicroscope with only topical anesthesia.

The use of diamond knives or sapphire blades has greatly improved the ease of surgery and postoperative predictability of incisional keratotomies. Astigmatic keratotomies are often employed for up to 6.0 D of astigmatism.

Corneal Wedge Additions

Wedge additions are used only for exceptionally high degrees of astigmatism, for example, in Terrien's marginal degeneration in which a relaxing incision is made and a donor cornea added to increase total corneal volume for tectonic support.

Disparate Diameter Graft Recipient Technique

This grafting method is done on virtually all transplants in which the diameter of the donor cornea is larger than that of the recipient. The graft promotes a tight fit, good wound coaptation, and a deepening of the anterior chamber to reduce chances of postoperative synechiae and glaucoma. It is only incidental that the increase in corneal curvature affects ultimate refractive error. An equal size recipient bed/donor tissue cut is occasionally used to reduce significant preoperative myopia.

Radial Keratotomy (RK)

In radial keratotomy, stromal incisions result in a peripheral corneal bulge and commensurate central flattening (Figure 6-6). With radial cuts to Descemet's membrane (approximately 90% to 95% of corneal

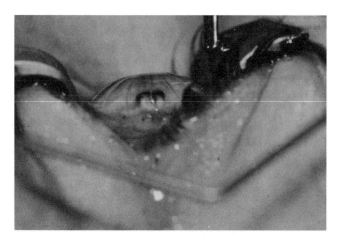

FIGURE 6-6 Significant corneal flattening with a compensatory bulge in the midperiphery is shown following 8-incision radial keratotomy. Recent findings suggest that the midperipheral cornea is actually flatter postoperatively than before surgery, with a significantly flatter central cornea.

thickness), the cornea is made weaker and intraocular pressure allows steepening of the peripheral cornea with associated central corneal flattening. This procedure was popularized by Sato et al. in 1953 in Japan. Initially, incisions were made from the endothelial surface. Needless to say, many of these patients have gone on to need penetrating keratoplasty. The Russian surgeon Fyodorov repopularized the technique using 16 anterior surface radial incisions. As a result of animal and human experimentation and technological advances, most surgery now requires only four to eight radial incisions. Routine complications include undercorrection and overcorrection of myopia.

Currently, radial keratotomy is considered fairly safe and effective, with as many as 90% of low myopes (<4.00 D) achieving an uncorrected visual acuity of 20/40 or better. Furthermore, fewer incisions and larger optic zones have lessened the likelihood of postoperative glare. Nonetheless, radial keratotomy is not without limitations. Approximately 15% to 20% of all RK patients will experience a long-term progressive hyperopic shift. Corneal microperforations also are common and a range of 5% to 10% corneal endothelial loss has been confirmed by numerous studies (Figure 6-7). Some patients report persistent glare or starburst effect, particularly while driving at night. There have been documented cases of endophthalmitis following RK. The long-term effect of reduced corneal tensile strength is debatable, but reports have demonstrated that subsequent blunt trauma can lead to corneal rupture.

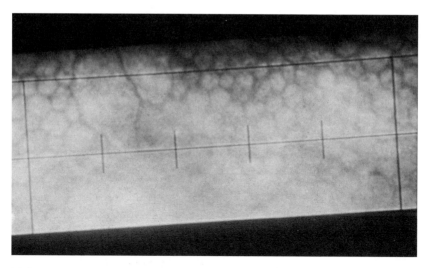

FIGURE 6-7 Endothelial morphology is obvious in this postincisional keratotomy patient. Polymegethism and pleomorphism are not uncommon with the significant cutting depth required to gain adequate flattening. (Courtesy B. Weiner).

Miscellaneous Techniques

Infant Donor Corneas

Keratometry of the newborn cornea reveals K readings in the range of 50 D to 55 D. The tissue is exceptionally elastic and difficult to work with. Using infant corneas has proven beneficial in correcting hyperopia and unilateral aphakia. The use of an infant donor cornea is a contraindication to insertion of an intraocular lens. Corneas less than 34 weeks old have induced myopia in aphakic recipients. A full-term cornea (that is, 40 weeks or older) usually produces results close to emmetropia in the aphakic eye. Donor corneas between 1 month and 1 year old correct approximately 50% of aphakic refractive error.

Thermokeratoplasty

Thermokeratoplasty entails the application of heat to shrink corneal collagen, thereby flattening the keratoconic cornea. The procedure was popularized in the 1970s by Gasset and Kaufman, but has fallen out of favor because of unpredictability, creation of basement membrane disorders, induction of stromal vascularization, and potential technical wound healing problems if penetrating keratoplasty is necessary. Subsequently, Rowsey et al rekindled interest in thermokeratoplasty with the use of the "Los Alamos keratoplasty." This procedure uses a radio frequency probe to shrink corneal collagen, thereby inducing controlled selective refractive changes. The procedure induces major scars outside the visual axis and is currently experimental.

Laser Thermokeratoplasty

The cobalt magnesium fluoride laser has shown promise in correcting myopia, hyperopia, and astigmatism in animal models. The central zone in myopic reduction is subject to much less energy when applied in a "halo" effect. This approach also has proven beneficial for treatment of low to moderate hyperopia. Whether applied in a central application or in an annular "halo" pattern, the stroma appears hazy immediately after surgery. This central stromal haze usually clears in 2 to 5 weeks.[16,17] Some controversy exists as to whether stromal rehydration will subsequently lead to refractive error regression.

Intrastromal Photoablation

Recent research has indicated that a double frequency Nd:YAG laser (picosecond laser) may be beneficial in performing intrastromal photoablation. This laser technology has already been studied for its efficacy in glaucoma therapy, including sclerostomy and iridotomy. In refractive surgery, the laser is focused at the cornea[1] midstroma and a tissue ablation is performed. The ablated stroma is subsequently resorbed with an attending collapse of anterior stroma onto the posterior stroma (Figure 6-8). This flattens the anterior corneal surface and reduces myopia.

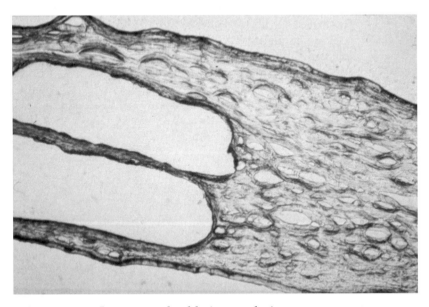

FIGURE 6-8 Intrastromal ablation techniques represent a new frontier in refractive surgery. A stromal "collapse" is expected, resulting in central corneal flattening.

Photorefractive Keratectomy (PRK)

Perhaps no refractive surgery technique has become more popular in recent years than PRK. The 193 nm argon-fluoride excimer laser has the potential to excise corneal tissue with micron accuracy, minimal collateral tissue damage, and an optically smooth surface. In this procedure, the corneal epithelium is removed and Bowman's membrane is exposed for laser ablation. The lasing is carried out in an en-face approach with approximately 40 μm to 100 μm of corneal tissue being removed. In the ensuing week the wound reepithelializes, and in the following 3 to 6 months the stroma remodels. PRK is best suited for the correction of mild to moderate myopia and astigmatism. Its efficacy in hyperopia is not well established. In the final analysis, PRK's accuracy and predictability is comparable to the most refined RK procedures. However, the risk of perforation, endophthalmitis, diurnal fluctuations in vision, progressive hyperopia, and globe rupture are eliminated. Decentered ablations, persistent stromal haze, central islands, and irregular astigmatism are infrequent sequelae to excimer PRK.

Intraocular Lens Implantation

The implantation of lenses after cataract extraction is a form of refractive surgery. With accurate keratometry and A-scan measurements, the pseudophakic patient is virtually assured of a predictable refractive outcome. Occasionally, a contact lens may be required if an improper lens power calculation is made, high astigmatism results, or an intraocular lens has to be removed.

Implanting intraocular lenses in phakic eyes is gaining popularity as a means of correcting ametropia while preserving accommodation. Early studies involving the Domilens (an anterior segment intraocular lens) were fraught with limitations, including endothelial touch. Current European studies employing anterior or posterior chamber intraocular lenses are demonstrating early favorable results.

Factors Affecting Predictability, Results, and Complications

Our understanding of factors affecting the outcome of refractive surgical procedures (whether related to the patient or the surgical technique) has come from the work of surgeons and from statistical analysis techniques such as multiple regression analysis.[1,3,6] Most of the comments in this section relate to results following RK, PRK, LASIK, and ALK (the procedures most often used today).

Several patient-related factors are important in eventual outcome of RK. These include patient age, sex, intraocular pressure, corneal diameter, and preoperative keratometry.[1,3,6] Older patients generally show more effect for the same amount of surgery than younger patients. Moreover, young women do not receive as much refractive effect as young men, although this difference tends to diminish with age. These differences could be related to hormonal influence on collagen.[1] The age-related increase in effect may be tied to an increase in scleral rigidity.[1,6]

Greater postoperative intraocular pressure results in a greater RK effect immediately following surgery. In addition, one can generally expect a greater effect with steeper corneas and larger corneal diameters.[1,4-6]

Surgical factors that will affect RK visual outcomes include optic zone size, incision length, and incision depth.[1] Secondary factors include peripheral redeepening and the number of incisions. Nomograms designed by a group or by a particular surgeon from multiregression analysis are based on results of a particular surgical technique. What may be appropriate or adequate for one surgeon may not translate well to another.

CLINICAL PEARL

Nomograms designed by a group or by a particular surgeon from multiregression analysis are based on results of a particular surgical technique. What may be appropriate or adequate for one surgeon may not translate well to another.

Modifiers are often needed to compensate for differences in surgical technique. Research by Dietz et al. has shown that most of RK's effects occur after the first four incisions. Surgeons may choose to redeepen surgical incisions. Although enhancements are an accepted form of retreatment, it is often wise to accept the results achieved after the first procedure and not redeepen or add to the number of the incisions. Lengthening incisions is a commonly used enhancement technique.

RK incisions heal much as other corneal incisions, through the process of avascular wound healing.[1] During the first 2 days, the epithelium slides into the incisions, forming an epithelial plug (Figure 6-9). During the next 2 weeks, the plugs are replaced by fibroblasts.[1,10,18-20] After 3 months the fibroblasts disappear. However, if plugs remain they may work their way to the surface while the patient is wearing contact lenses and rupture, thereby increasing the risk of infectious keratitis. This is particularly important for those individuals who undergo enhancement procedures in which existing incisions are reopened. The potential for incision epithelial plugs increases under these circumstances.

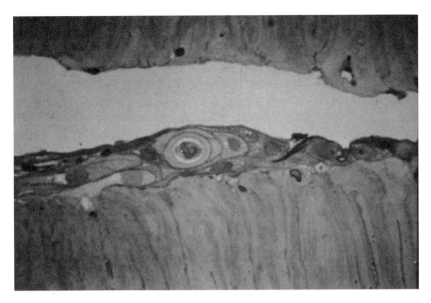

FIGURE 6-9   Epithelial inclusion plugs resulting from poor irrigation technique or faulty blades will gradually work their way to the anterior corneal surface, increasing the risk of infectious keratitis.

Endothelial cell loss appears to have little effect on the outcome of contact lens wear. However, it is prudent to use a high flux material whenever possible. Recent studies show no progressive cell loss following RK.[1]

In excimer laser PRK, patient variables such as sex, age, corneal curvature and thickness, and intraocular pressure have a significantly smaller impact on surgical outcome. The degree of myopia reduction and the ablation zone's diameter determine the amount of stromal photoablation; this may ultimately influence the results. In excimer PRK, the epithelium is removed and photoablation begins at Bowman's membrane. In the first 1 to 4 days postoperatively, epithelial regeneration and migration fills in the surgical defect. At this point, the epithelium may be thickened and irregular. During the next 6 months the epithelium returns to normal. The underlying stroma remains relatively dormant until approximately 1 month postoperatively. At this time, stromal keratocyte activation results in a fine anterior stromal haze. As the stroma remodels, a refractive regression ensues. Ultimately, the anterior stromal haze regresses by 6 to 12 months postoperatively. Controversy persists regarding the efficacy of postoperative topical steroid use in modulating wound healing, including stromal haze and refractive outcome. Current experience indicates that postoperative topical steroids can influence refractive outcome, but have little influence on stromal haze.

PRK is a more refined procedure than RK from an accuracy and predictability standpoint. Undoubtedly, less likelihood exists of progressive hyperopic shift and diurnal refractive fluctuations in PRK. However, interpatient variability in wound healing influences outcome in PRK. Persistent stromal haze, elevated central islands, decentered ablations, and irregular astigmatism have obscured an otherwise successful PRK procedure for some individuals. Many of these complications can be effectively treated by a "tincture of time." A reablation may be necessary for resolving some of these issues; however, fewer than 5% of all PRK patients require additional surgery. This compares favorably with the 15% to 25% enhancement rate commonly associated with RK.

Significant long-term follow-up data is lacking for patients who have undergone ALK and LASIK. Because the microkeratome dissects the cornea at anterior one-third stromal depth without epithelial involvement, the postoperative course appears cleaner than with PRK. Often the cornea appears normal the day after ALK and LASIK, with the exception of circumferential incision. The thickened irregular epithelium and anterior stromal haze commonly associated with postoperative PRK are absent in ALK and LASIK. Furthermore, because the microkeratome incision is through the anterior stroma, the eye does not manifest the compromised integrity seen in RK.

Despite the many appealing aspects of ALK and LASIK, some problems remain. A potential exists for corneal cap misalignment with associated irregular astigmatism. An inaccurate microkeratome pass can result in significant residual ametropia. Despite these shortcomings, ALK and LASIK can significantly reduce higher degrees of myopia. ALK and LASIK is currently recognized as a procedure for reducing myopia of greater than 16 D, with a predictability of $+/-$ 2 D.

Postoperative Care and Complications

In most refractive procedures, including RK, PRK, LASIK, and ALK, certain postoperative side effects are fairly predictable. If a clinician follows appropriate postoperative patient care protocols, complications are rare. However, there are caveats to consider.

Bandaging is often necessary, depending on the procedure. Following PRK and "capless" ALK, a bandage lens is crucial to aid reepithelialization (Figure 6-10). Collagen may aid wound healing,[21,22] and collagen gels have been shown to maintain corneal epithelial cells in vitro.

Fyodorov et al. have reported the beneficial results of the collagen shield application following RK.[21] Aquavella et al. have studied the efficacy of a corneal collagen shield on epithelial and stromal wound healing in rabbits following eight incision RK.[21] A significant difference between treated and untreated corneas was noted. At 8 hours, specimens fixed for light and electron microscopy showed more

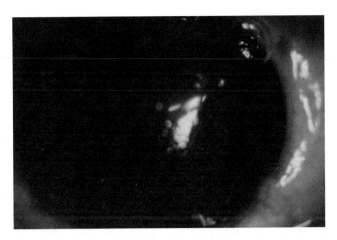

FIGURE 6-10 A corneal shield made of collagen has been placed on a cornea to promote healing following epikeratoplasty.

complete epithelial healing in the treated eye than in the untreated eye.[21] At 24 hours, the number and distribution of surface epithelial microvilli were more normal in the treated eye. Stromal lamellae in the treated cornea were more regular, with less edema at the wound site, limited keratocyte reaction, and fewer polymorphonuclear cells[21] (Figure 6-11).

Because the dissolution of soluble collagen is related to the protolytic enzyme reaction, the lid closure mechanism must not cause irritation and increased tearing.[21] Reduced stromal edema may be a simple mechanical protective effect, or may relate to the effect of hydrolyzed dissociation products of collagen. Collagen may absorb collagenase or attract neutrophils, an additional benefit.[22]

Collagen lenses have been used following virtually all forms of refractive surgery to advance healing and bridge incisions with new connective tissue. Often a collagen lens is applied followed by an appropriate hydrogel lens in a piggyback fashion. Collagen has two times the oxygen permeability of traditional hydrogel lenses; this increases exponentially as collagen dissolves, usually over a 12 to 24 hour period depending on the material's thickness and cross-linkage characteristics. There should be little problem with oxygen flux.[22] Even if the shield decenters, it remains in colloidal suspension and will probably aid healing. After this shield dissolves, the bandage hydrogel is left in place for protection. In many cases the hydrogel lens remains until complete epithelialization occurs. This shield often helps ease dryness after surgery by providing simple lubrication.

The deliverance of water-soluble topical drugs to the anterior segment using collagen shields has worked reasonably well, with results equivalent to those achieved by injection.[23] Antibiotics, steroids, and certain glaucoma medications may be delivered to the eye

A

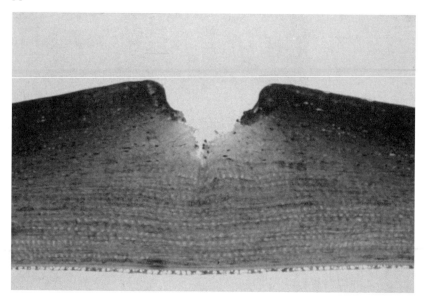

B

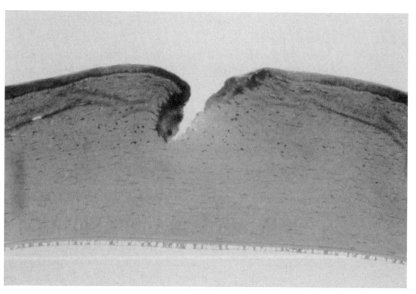

FIGURE 6-11 Collagen has been shown to enhance healing follow-ing 8-incision radial keratotomy in rabbits. More edema, less differentiated epithelium and more reactive keratocytes are shown in the untreated eye **(A)** versus the treated eye **(B)**.

by this route. This provides a reservoir without patching or applying additional drops. Little need remains to use preserved eye drops.

Some controversy persists as to whether the eye should be patched with steri-strips[1] after RK and other surface area techniques. Advocates of the open-eye approach feel that patching does not sufficiently enhance reepithelialization over the incision site. Additionally, a patched environment provides a potential for infection. A recent phenomenon seen is anterior stromal infiltrates in the short-term postoperative phase of PRK patients. Although these infiltrates do not appear to be infectious, they are most often associated with the use of topical nonsteroidal antiinflammatory agents in conjunction with a hydrophilic bandage lens.

The postoperative course of a typical refractive surgery patient often is uncomplicated. Most patients can be appropriately managed with very few drugs or manipulations. When combined with proper patient education, the postoperative course in refractive keratoplasty can be extremely uneventful.

However, lack of attention to the basic mechanics of wound healing and corneal immune barriers will assuredly result in potentially dangerous complications.[1] Complications following these procedures include overcorrection, undercorrection, induced irregular astigmatism,[21,24] corneal perforation, postoperative glare, fluctuation in refraction,[25,26] decreased night acuity, photophobia, reduced best-corrected acuity,[26,27] monocular diplopia, multiple ghost images, need for reoperation, recurrent corneal erosions, and inability to wear contact lenses. Further complications include iron lines, neovascularization, scarring, epithelial inclusion cysts, optic atrophy,[28] exacerbation of corneal dystrophy, endothelial cell loss, glaucoma, cataracts, infection, vitreous wick syndrome, iritis, retinal detachment, decreased corneal sensitivity, and endophthalmitis.[1,29-32] Of course, many changes are benign (such as iron lines that are caused by tear redistribution with epithelial irregularity and erosion).

Patients who have experienced adverse effects may be reluctant to proceed with surgery on the fellow eye, highlighting another problem. Implicit in the decision to undergo refractive surgery in most instances is the acceptance of the need for bilateral surgery to avoid anisometropia.[7] It is prudent to simulate uncorrected residual refractive error and monovision effects by first fitting the surgical candidate with contact lenses. For some individuals this is the only way they can fully understand the benefits and limitations of refractive surgery.

This is another area in which contact lenses for anisometropia or astigmatism are needed. Anisometropia with associated aniseikonia and compromised depth perception are present in many of these patients.[3] Several case series have demonstrated a shift toward more plus,[3-5,32,33] often several years after RK and other surface area techniques. In working with these patients, the clinician should anticipate some difficulty because of altered corneal topography[34] and morphology, and because of psychosocial reasons.[7] Contact lens application for these disappointed and frustrated patients will often result in failure.

Corneal onlay procedures have demonstrated complications during both short-term and long-term postoperative phases. After interfacial scarring, graft extrusion and infection are the most frequently encountered problems.[35-37] Persistent epithelial defects and vascularization also are common. If vascularization occurs in an eye that may later require full thickness grafting, one must also be concerned about an increased antigen load and subsequent rejection.[38]

Generally about 5% to 6% of all epikeratoplasty lenticules are removed.[35,38] If a lenticule is removed and a keratectomy performed, unpredictable results can occur depending on how the wound heals. For example, there can be a reduced amount of myopia because of corneal flattening.

Experiments have been conducted on augmentation effects following considerable undercorrection. These included the use of systemic medications that either increase intraocular pressure or affect collagen cross-linkage.[1] Unfortunately, these medications also can be cytotoxic. Any procedure performed after the initial incisions have been made is sometimes unpredictable.

When used immediately after surgery, thicker hydrogel lenses have proven beneficial in enhancing incisional keratotomies and lessening myopia.[39] Unfortunately, other experiments have shown that when a hydrogel lens is fit in the early postoperative course, an increase in neovascularization occurs (Plate 23).

The extra thickness in the periphery of a minus lens induces peripheral corneal swelling and a secondary central corneal flattening. Because hydration differs between the central and peripheral cornea, different collagen spacing and nerve innervation differences may account for this phenomenon. Even with uniform swelling of the central and peripheral cornea, the radius of curvature will increase, with a net effect of decreased myopia.

Contrast sensitivity testing in surface area techniques is another interesting issue. A decrease in function generally occurs, especially at low illumination levels.[27] Pupil size and new shape factors probably account for this complication.

Contact Lens Indications and Fitting Principles Following Surgery

Fortunately, the most common complications following refractive surgery are overcorrection, undercorrection and irregular astigmatism.[3] All of these generally require contact lenses for correction, especially in cases of anisometropia in which the patient has elected to not undergo a second eye procedure. Severe complications such as cataract formation, corneal infection, and endophthalmitis are rare.

Most optical complications are caused by technical problems during the procedure. For example, in RK too many incisions may have been made, or there may be a decentered optic zone or incisional incursion beyond the optic zone. Inclusion cysts, wide scars secondary to redeepening procedures, and astigmatic procedures at an incorrect axis also may lead to complications[3] (Plate 24). In PRK, complications include irregular astigmatism, decentered ablations, central islands, and stromal haze (Plate 25).

Fitting a contact lens after refractive surgery carries a reduced success rate for practical and psychosocial reasons. The topography has undergone hysteresis and is often irregular. Reduced endothelial cell function and a disrupted tear film may result. Acuity is often unstable and unpredictable, especially with hydrogel lenses. Corneal rigidity accounts for the less than ideal results that may occur. Arrowsmith et al found 40% to 60% of their RK patients had at least 1 D of residual refractive error.[6,33]

Early literature demonstrates that approximately 30% to 70% of RK procedures require substantial correction for residual refractive error, often necessitating contact lenses.[3,33,40,41] Recent advances in RK have undoubtedly reduced these percentages; however, some still require postoperative contact lenses. Current research suggests that 2% to 4% of RK patients opt for contact lens correction, although many more might actually benefit from contact lens wear. Contact lenses usually offer a predictable means of achieving best corrected visual acuity and eliminate the need for additional surgery if any residual refractive error remains. However, certain considerations remain in fitting the patient who has undergone a surface area technique such as RK.

CLINICAL PEARL

Current research suggests that 2% to 4% of RK patients opt for contact lens correction, although many more might actually benefit from contact lens wear.

Fitting goals are similar regardless of the surgical procedure employed. Important considerations include lens centration, nearly equal distribution of lens mass across the cornea, minimal rocking in the horizontal meridian, and minimal bearing in zonal areas[41] (Plate 26).

Patients with marked limbal injection, severe vascularization, significant corneal staining or edema, corneal deformation, rejection episode, or anterior chamber reaction should not be fitted with contact lenses. Corneal sensitivity is greatly reduced during the immediate postoperative period,[42] and care must be given to early contact lens application. The lens should only be fitted after corneal edema clears.[33,40] It generally takes as long as 6 months before corneal edema clears completely. If the lens is fitted too early, severe fluctuations in vision may result. It is often difficult to achieve good centration with contact lenses on these patients. With almost any lens that exhibits limbal override, lens comfort will be compromised regardless of the material used. An additional concern with lens decentration is exposure staining that may be closer to visual axis than normally seen with 3 to 9 o'clock staining.

Clinicians making an initial lens selection will consider keratometry readings following surgery. These may be misleading because diurnal fluctuations are common. They also give the fitter little information about the midperipheral and far peripheral corneal areas.[34,41,43] In RK, the cornea generally grows steeper throughout the day because of arteriole pulse that distends the globe[25] or because of steroid use following surgery. Diurnal variation usually stops in 2 or 3 months,[25] but can go on for many years, especially with prolonged postoperative steroid use. In PRK, corneal topography is essentially unchanged outside the ablation zone and diurnal variation is minimal.

El Hage has described fitting RK patients in a quasi-ortho-keratology modality to augment undercorrection and further flatten the cornea,[41] beyond the surgical effects. He found the cornea's peripheral portion to be 3 D to 4 D steeper than the central cornea after RK. This occasionally requires the use of peripheral curves steeper than the base curve. Diameters can range from 8 mm to 12 mm, optic zones of 6 mm to 8 mm, and peripheral curves 1 D to 5 D steeper than the base curve.

Forstat found that patients who had been overcorrected following RK in an attempt to alter topography were successfully fitted much steeper (as much as 10 D) than postoperative k readings. These ortho-keratology patients held at about 1.5 D of correction. A greater effect was found with corneas that were fitted less than a year after surgery, and those that had more than eight incisions.[44] Caroline suggests placing four fixation dots 4 mm from the edge of the keratometer opening, and using these fixation points to determine midperipheral keratometry.[45] He feels these midperipheral readings (3 mm from the fixation) are crucial in determining base curve and peripheral curve radii. Davis advocates a monocurve design, gaspermeable lens fitted 3 D to 4 D flatter than preoperative keratometry to minimize bearing and decentration. Similarly, Janes used 9.5 mm diameter Polycon lenses, and reduced the diameter appropriately to allow a steeper peripheral curve system.[41]

Several special design RK lenses now exist. Four recently released designs—the OK-60 (Contex Inc.), Ni-Cone (Lancaster Contact Lens), Menicon Plateau (Menicon), and RK-Bridge (Conforma) lenses—seem ideal for these patients. Bearing areas should be 1.5 mm to 2.0 mm

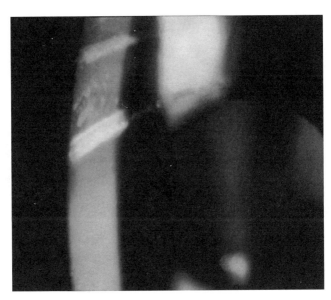

FIGURE 6-12 Areas of basement membrane changes may persist if the epithelium has been "squeezed" or violated following cross-incisions. This can complicate contact lens wear. Fortunately, few of these procedures are done today.

distal to the central zone with 1 mm wide bands whenever possible. Corneal changes because of a malpositioned Bowman's membrane, immature hemidesmosomes, and asymmetric wound healing can further complicate this approach.[10,19] Certain corneal areas have the potential to stain indefinitely (Figure 6-12).

Base curves are best chosen by lens evaluation, with a base curve slightly flatter than the presurgical k reading as a starting point, and using more plus than the preoperative spherical equivalent.[45-47] If this information is unavailable, the clinician should obtain keratometry readings from the fellow eye if no surgery has been done there. Unfortunately, Ackley found that only 40% of RK patients had preoperative keratometry. Some researchers advocate a prerefractive surgery diagnostic contact lens fitting as a template in case postsurgical contact lenses are necessary.

In evaluating base curve, modifications may be made based upon slit lamp evaluation of the fit. If too much movement is evident, a steeper base curve or larger diameter is usually appropriate. Alternately, if there is not enough movement the base curve can be flattened or the diameter decreased. In general, peripheral curves are chosen relative to lens position and diameter. They should not be steep enough to obstruct movement, nor flat enough to prevent proper tear venting.[36] Secondary curves at least 3.5 D steeper than the base curve exert a greater contouring effect.

A   **B**

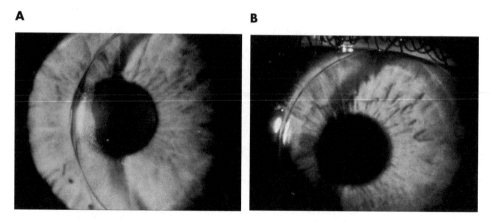

FIGURE 6-13 **A,** Lens decentration is not uncommon with lens application following radial keratotomy. **B,** Prism may aid centration, as shown in this case.

Decentration is another common problem that requires lens modification. If the lenses ride high, a change in diameter and base curve may help. Adding prism may allow the lens to assume a more inferior position because of increased lens mass (Figure 6-13). If the lens rides low, a lighter material (higher index of refraction) with lower specific gravity may help. The use of a myoflange along with diameter or base curve change also may be helpful. Increasing lens diameter does not always aid lens centration because transition zones may have been altered after surgery.[41]

Almost any rigid gas-permeable lens will show central pooling after RK. If excessively poor tear exchange and bubble formation occurs, they may result in edema, especially with low-oxygen materials. Flatter base curves or fenestrations may help. Smaller optic zones also may control undesirable bearing relationships.

Contact lenses tend to center over the cornea's steepest part and therefore do not often center well after RK. Preoperative shapes usually resemble prolate ellipses. After the surgery, the shape becomes an oblate ellipse with a knee effect in the midperiphery.[4]

Generally, optic zones should be relatively small, although large diameters are often used. This provides better control of peripheral curve effects, as in keratoconus, in which topography is opposite to that in RK. The downside to small optic zones is the potential for glare (especially at night).

Corneal topography is a new technology that is essential in the preoperative and postoperative evaluation of refractive surgery patients. Many of these devices employ reflective photokeratoscopy, in which a multiple ring reflected image is scanned, digitized, and converted to an interactive dioptric map[43] (Plate 27). Other topography instruments are available, including a stereography technique

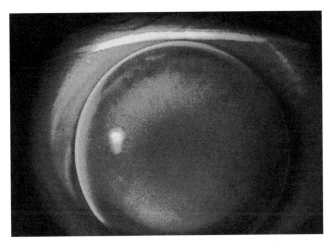

FIGURE 6-14 Good centration of a contact lens is shown on a cornea following excimer laser ablation. Central pooling is expected, along with reasonably good alignment in the far midperiphery and periphery, because the ablation zone is relatively small (5 mm).

employing vertical rasters by Par Technology and another device by Orbtek that uses a slit image rather than Placido rings.

Spherical overrefraction with a rigid gas-permeable lens generally satisfies visual requirements. If residual astigmatism from contact lens flexure or lenticular astigmatism persists, appropriate modifications can be made in contact lens center thickness, base curve selection, or prescription.

Fortunately, the post-PRK patient is often easier to fit than the RK patient. The central 5 mm to 6 mm ablated cornea has been flattened, but the midperiphery and periphery are unaltered. The patient's preoperative lens worn before laser surgery is often sufficient. A slight power change (usually less minus power) is often appropriate. Generally, standard design rigid gas-permeable lenses work well with a slight apical clearance flourescein pattern or an aligned fluorescein pattern with slight edge lift (Figure 6-14). Hydrogel lenses can be used for long-term management of residual refractive error or as a surgical adjunct in PRK. In the latter case hydrogel lenses are used for patients who demonstrate minimal healing as evidenced by little haze and persistent hyperopia. In these cases a hydrogel lens can modulate wound healing by stimulating the healing response.

Complications

In one large case series of RK, 48% of eyes fitted with hydrogel lenses developed neovascularization.[40] In contrast, only two eyes fitted with rigid gas-permeable lenses developed neovascularization.[33,40] Usually neovascularization is superficial along the radial incision lines. Because incisions are no longer placed through the limbal sulcus, decreased scarring occurs. With decreased scarring, better blades, and shorter and fewer incisions the incidence of advanced neovascularization has decreased.[9] Extended-wear hydrogel lenses should never be considered because of the risk of severe neovascularization. It is prudent to use rigid gas-permeable lenses whenever possible, because hydrogel, hybrid (e.g., SoftPerm), and piggyback systems also can cause significant neovascularization.

CLINICAL PEARL

Extended-wear hydrogel lenses should never be considered because of the risk of severe neovascularization.

Recurrent corneal erosion also is possible, and often a transient basement membrane change occurs after surgery (Figure 6-15). Inclusion cysts along the incisions sites also have been described. Problems in fitting hydrogel lenses (in addition to neovascularization) include poor optical quality because of topographical changes and tear effects from pooling. Lens compression over this area can occur with rigid gas-permeable lenses. Centration over the visual axis may be a problem, especially with lenses with small optic zones. Often lenses decenter downward and outward and excessive movement occurs. Regression following RK also has occurred.[6]

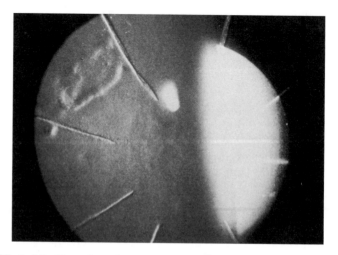

FIGURE 6-15 Transient basement membrane changes may follow radial keratotomy and cause recurrent corneal erosions because of poor epithelial adhesion ("leaky Epithelium Syndrome").

There seems to be a central corneal steepening following rigid lens wear. This is most likely caused by corneal contouring to the contact lens' back surface.

A direct correlation was never found between k readings and spectacle refraction after this procedure. Usually a greater spectacle effect is seen than can be documented by keratometry readings.

As soon as peripheral corneal edema resolves (usually after 6 months), hydrogel daily-wear lenses can be successfully employed, with caution, when needed.

In fitting lenses after therapeutic lamellar onlay (epikeratoplasty), surface reepithelialization is a major problem.[42,46-49] Theoretically, the lenticule can be removed, but corneal steepening has been documented with aphakic and myopic patients.

Keratectomy is not often performed anymore. It is occasionally performed, however, to refine the area where the onlay will be applied. A wing effect is often seen in certain areas of the midperipheral cornea, especially if a keratectomy is not performed. This wing effect has been documented by corneal mapping devices. This may be a difficult area to fit because of the myopic lenticule's raised wings.[47]

Lembach and others have concluded that the majority of epikeratoplasty procedures performed for keratoconus achieve satisfactory visual results with spectacles or contact lenses.[48] However, patients requiring contact lenses should be closely monitored for vascularization and scarring.[49]

Some of these patients will have to be grafted; they should be closely monitored for vascular changes. Hydrogel lenses are used initially as a bandage, with or without collagen. This allows for reepithelialization. They will remain in place for several weeks, with myopic epikeratoplasty patients requiring a much flatter fit for the central zone. With keratoconus and aphakic epikeratoplasty patients, steeper base curves usually are required. Again, vascularization with the use of hydrogel lenses is a major concern and must be closely monitored, because a tendency toward interfacial scarring exists.

Light sensitivity and glare may be worse in contact lens wearers who undergo refractive surgery. If contact lenses cannot successfully be worn, or if they do not improve acuity, full-thickness penetrating keratoplasty may be needed to restore vision following these refractive procedures.[38]

Conclusion

It is not uncommon to encounter disappointment and frustration in patients who choose to wear contact lenses following refractive surgery. Refractive corneal surgery is a new, exciting, but still evolving field. Current procedures are constantly evolving and improving, and optical complications are concomitantly decreasing.

With a better understanding of corneal wound healing, optical complications following refractive surgical procedures should continue to decline. Until all optical problems have been resolved, contact lens therapy should continue to be a therapeutic mainstay.

References

1. Sanders DR, Hoffman RF (ed): *Refractive Surgery: A Text of Radial Keratotomy*, Thorofare, New Jersey, 1985, Slack Publishers.
2. Maguire LJ : Refractive surgery, success, and public health, *Am J Ophthalmol* 117:394-396, 1994.
3. Binder PS: Optical problems following refractive surgery, *Ophthalmol* 93:739, 1986.
4. Santos VR, Waring GO, et al: Relationship between refractive error and visual acuity in the pre-operative evaluation of radial keratotomy (PERK) study, *Arch Ophthalmol* 105:86-92, 1987.
5. Lynn MJ, Waring GO, Sperduto RD: Factors affecting outcome and predictability of radial keratotomy in the PERK study, *Arch Ophthalmol* 105:42-57, 1987.
6. Arrowsmith PN, Marks RG: Visual, refractive, and keratometric results of radial keratotomy (five year follow-up), *Arch Ophthalmol* 107:506-511, 1989.
7. Powers ME, et al: Psychosocial findings in radial keratotomy patients two years after surgery, *Ophthalmol* 91:1193-1198, 1984.
8. Erickson D: Psychosocial characteristics of patients having refractive surgery, Paper: The National Research Symposium On Contact Lenses, Anaheim, August 1992.
9. O'Day DM: Visual impairment following radial keratotomy: A cluster of cases, *Ophthalmol* 93:319-326, 1986.
10. Fyodorov SN, Durnev VV: Operation of dosaged dissection of corneal arcuate ligament in cases of myopia of mild degree, *Ann Ophthalmol* 11:1485-1490, 1979.
11. Nichols BD, Williams PA, Spigelman AV, Lindstrom RL: Epikeratophakia: Technique, modification and visual results compared to the national study, *J Cataract Refract Surg* 15:312-316, 1989.
12. Binder PS: The excimer laser and radial keratotomy: two vastly different approaches for myopia correction, *Arch Ophthalmol* 108:1541-1542, 1990.
13. Seiler T, Wollensack J: Myopic photorefractive keratectomy with the excimer laser, *Ophthalmol* 98:1156-1163, 1991.
14. Bettman J, Tennenhouse D: Medicolegal aspects in ophthalmology, *Int Ophthalmol Clin* 20:33-42, 1980.
15. Notz, R: Personal communication, 1986.
16. Marmer RH: Thermal keratoplasty confirmed effective as a refractive error treatment, *Ophthalmol Times* 14:3, 1989.
17. Rowsey JA: Laser thermokeratoplasty shows promise, *Ophthalmol Times* 14:4, 1989.
18. Shivitz IR, Arrowsmith PN: Delayed keratitis after radial keratotomy, *Arch Ophthalmol* 104:1153-1155, 1986.
19. Glasgow BJ, Brown HH, et al: Traumatic dehiscence of incisions seven years after radial keratotomy, *Am J Ophthalmol* 106:703-707, 1988.
20. Insler MS, Sample HC: Delayed microbial keratitis following radial keratotomy, *CLAO* 14:163-164, 1988.
21. Aquavella JV, delCerro M, et al: The effect of collagen bandage lens on corneal wound healing, *Ophthalmol Surg* 18:570-573, 1987.
22. Sawusch M, O'Brien T, et al: The collagen corneal shield, *Am J Ophthalmol* 106:279-281, 1988.
23. Kaufman H: Collagen shield drug delivery, *CLAO* 15:178, 1989.
24. McDonnell PJ, Caroline PJ, Salz J: Irregular astigmatism after radial and astigmatic keratotomy, *Am J Ophthalmol* 107:42-46, 1989.

25. MacRae S, Rich L, et al: Diurnal variation in vision after radial keratotomy, *Am J Ophthalmol* 107:262-267, 1989.
26. Santos VR, Waring Go, et al: Morning to evening change in refraction, corneal curvature and visual acuity four years after radial keratotomy in the PERK study, *Ophthalmol* 95:1487-1493, 1988.
27. Krasnow MM, Avetison SE, et al: The effect of radial keratotomy on contrast sensitivity, *Am J Ophthalmol* 105:651-654, 1988.
28. Jindra LF: Blindness following retrobulbar anesthesia for astigmatic keratotomy, *Ophthalmol Surg* 20:433-435, 1989.
29. Robin JP, Beatty RF, et al: *Mycobacterium chelonei* keratitis after radial keratotomy, *Am J Ophthalmol* 102:72-79, 1986.
30. DePaolis MD, Aquavella JV, Shovlin JP: Post surgical contact lens management. In: Silbert JA (ed.): *Anterior Segment Complications of Contact Lens Wear,* New York, 1994, Churchill Livingstone.
31. Bourque LB, Lynn MJ, Waring GO, et al: Spectacle and contact lens wear 6 years after radial keratotomy in the PERK study, *Ophthalmol* 101:421-431, 1994.
32. Waring GO, Lynn MJ, McDonnell PJ, et al: Results of the prospective evaluation of radial keratotomy (PERK) study 10 years after surgery, *Arch Ophthalmol* 112:1298-1308, 1994.
33. Shivitz IA: Contact lenses in the treatment of patients with over-corrected radial keratotomy, *Ophthalmol* 94:899, 1987.
34. McDonnell PJ, Garbus J, Lopez PF; Topographic analysis and visual acuity after radial keratotomy, *Am J Ophthalmol* 106:1224-1227, 1988.
35. Binder PS, Zavala EY: Why do some epikeratoplasties fail?, *Arch Ophthalmol* 105:63-69, 1987.
36. Beekhuis WH, McCarey BE, et al: Complications of hydrogel intracorneal lenses in monkeys, *Arch Ophthalmol* 105:116-122, 1989.
37. Shovlin JP: The use of alloplastics: a new realm of refractive surgery?, *Int Cont Lens Clin* 16:304-306, 1989.
38. Frantz JM, Limber MB, et al: Penetrating keratoplasty after epikeratophakia for keratoconus, *Arch Ophthalmol* 106:1224-1227, 1988.
39. Edwards GA: Corneal flattening associated with daily soft contact lenses following radial keratotomy, *J Refract Surg* 3:54, 1987.
40. Shivitz IR: Fitting contact lenses after radial keratotomy, *Cont Lens Forum* 13:38-39, 1988.
41. Shovlin JP, Kame RT, et al: How to fit an irregular cornea, *Rev Optom* 124:88-98, 1987.
42. Shivitz IR, Arrowsmith PN: Corneal sensitivity after radial keratotomy, *Ophthalmol* 95:827-835, 1988.
43. Ghormley DJ, Gersten M, et al: Corneal modeling, *Cornea* 7:30-38, 1988.
44. Prescriber's Panel, Paragon Optical, Meza, Arizona, 1988.
45. Ackley KD, Caroline PJ, Davis LJ: Retrospective evaluation of rigid gas permeable contact lenses on radial keratotomy patients, *Optom Vis Sci (suppl.)* 70:32-37, 1993.
46. Aquavella JV, Shovlin JP, Pascucci SE, DePaolis MD: How contact lenses fit into refractive surgery, *Rev Ophthalmol* 1:36-39, 1994.
47. Gusto J: Contact lens fitting after myopic keratomileusis, *Trans Br Cont Lens Assoc, Int Cont Lens Cent Cong* 74:44-45, 1988.
48. Lembach RG, Lass JH, et al: The use of contact lenses after keratoconus epikeratoplasty, *Arch Ophthalmol* 107:364-368, 1989.
49. McDonald M, Kaufman HE, et al: Epikeratophakia for keratoconus, *Arch Ophthalmol* 104:1294-1300, 1986.

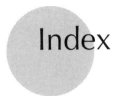

Index

Page numbers in *italic type* refer to figures. Tables are indicated by *t* following the page number.

A

Adherence, of contact lenses, with keratoconus, 10, *11*
Adults, young; *see* Young adults
Age
  IOL implantation and, 70-71
  RK outcome and, 148
ALK; *see* Lamellar keratoplasty, automated
Allograft rejection, of corneal grafts, 102, 104, *105*
Anesthesia, for keratoplasty, 99
Anisometropia
  refractive surgery and, 153
  surgery for, 140-41
Anterior chambers, flat, after cataract extraction, 72, *73*
Antibiotics
  delivered through collagen shields, 151, 153
  topical, with therapeutic soft contact lenses, 57, 64-65
Aphakia; *see also* Cataract extractions
  clinical evaluation of, 76-77, *78*
  contact lens applications in, 67-93
    cataract extraction complications during, 74-76, *76*
    children with, 87-88, *88*
    complications with, 89-92
    extended wear, 85-86
    geriatric patients and, 85-86, 89-90
    hydrogel contact lenses, 81, 82-84, 84*t*
      contraindications for, 83
    lens construction, 78-79, *79*
    magnification, 70
    mechanical problems, 78-82, *81*
    PMMA and, 80
    rigid contact lenses, 80-82, *81*
    UV filters, 92
    young adults with, 88-89, *90*

Aphakia—cont'd
  geriatric patients with
    contact lens applications in, 85-86, 89-90
    problems of, 84-86
  keratophakia for, 140
  optical correction for, 69-70
  pediatric
    contact lens applications in, 77, 87-88, *88*
    epikeratoplasty for, 140, *141*
Apical clearance lenses, for keratoconus, 30, *31*
Aspheric lenses, for keratoconus, 30-31
Astigmatism
  against-the-rule
    after cataract extraction, 77
    aphakic contact lens applications and, 80-81
  aphakic contact lens applications and, 80-81, 83
  causing reduced visual acuity, with keratoconus, 46
  oblique, with keratoconus, 23
  postkeratoplasty, 111
    surgical reduction of, 111-12, *112*
  reduction of
    with RGP lenses, 15
    surgery for, 111-12, *112*, 142, *143*, 146, 147
Atopic disease, causing keratoconus, 22
Attitudes, of postkeratoplasty patients, contact lens fitting and, 112-13

B

Bandage contact lenses, 53-65
  in bullous keratopathy, 57*t*, 57-58
  complications with, 63*t*, 63-64
  for corneal perforations, 61-62
  for damaged corneal epithelium, 53
  disposable, 55

165